CULTIVATING HEALTH

CULTIVATING HEALTH

CULTURAL PERSPECTIVES ON PROMOTING HEALTH

Edited by

Malcolm MacLachlan

*Trinity College,
University of Dublin,
Ireland*

JOHN WILEY & SONS, LTD
Chichester · New York · Weinheim · Brisbane · Singapore · Toronto

Copyright © 2001 by John Wiley & Sons Ltd,
Baffins Lane, Chichester,
West Sussex PO19 1UD, England

National   01243 779777
International   (+44) 1243 779777
e-mail (for orders and customer service enquiries):
cs-books@wiley.co.uk
Visit our Home Page on http://www.wiley.co.uk
or http://www.wiley.com

Other Wiley Editorial Offices

John Wiley & Sons, Inc., 605 Third Avenue,
New York, NY 10158-0012, USA

WILEY-VCH Verlag GmbH, Pappelallee 3,
D-69469 Weinheim, Germany

Jacaranda Wiley Ltd, 33 Park Road, Milton,
Queensland 4064, Australia

John Wiley & Sons (Asia) Pte Ltd, 2 Clementi Loop #02-01,
Jin Xing Distripark, Singapore 129809

John Wiley & Sons (Canada) Ltd, 22 Worcester Road,
Rexdale, Ontario M9W 1L1, Canada

Library of Congress Cataloging-in-Publication Data
Cultivating health : cultural perspectives on promoting health / edited by Malcolm MacLachlan.
    p. cm.
    Includes bibliographical references and index.
    ISBN 0-471-97725-X (cloth : alk. paper)
    1. Health promotion–Cross-cultural studies. 2. Health promotion. I. MacLachlan,
Malcolm.

RA427.8.C84 2000
613–dc21

00-043549

British Library Cataloguing in Publication Data

A catalogue record for this book is available from the British Library

ISBN 0 471 97725 X

Typeset in 10/12pt Palatino by Dorwyn Ltd, Rowlands Castle, Hants.
Printed and bound in Great Britain by Bookcraft (Bath) Ltd, Midsomer Norton, Somerset.
This book is printed on acid-free paper responsibly manufactured from sustainable forestry,
in which at least two trees are planted for each one used for paper production.

To

Eilish, Lara and Tess

CONTENTS

ABOUT THE EDITOR

Malcolm MacLachlan *Department of Psychology, Trinity College, University of Dublin, Ireland*

Malcolm MacLachlan is Senior Lecturer in Clinical & Health Psychology and a Fellow of Trinity College Dublin, the Psychological Society of Ireland and the Royal Anthropological Institute. He has the unintentional distinction of having degrees from universities in Scotland, England, Ireland and Wales. After completing his clinical psychology training at the Institute of Psychiatry, he has worked as a clinician, consultant in health service development and lecturer, in Europe and Africa. His major interests are in, *embodiment*, the interplay between culture and health and the organization of international aid. He has published numerous papers, authored two books—*Culture & Health* (Wiley 1997) and *Psychology of Aid* (Routledge 1998)—and edited several volumes, including the forthcoming *Cultivating Pluralism* (Oak Tree Press 2000).

ABOUT THE AUTHORS

Alastair Ager *Centre for International Health Studies,*
Queen Margaret University College, Edinburgh EH12 8TS, UK

Alastair Ager is Director of the Centre for International Health Studies and Professor of Applied Psychology at Queen Margaret University College, Edinburgh, and a research Associate of the Refugee Studies Programme, University of Oxford. He is a graduate of the universities of Keele, Wales and Birmingham. He has over fifty publications, spanning the fields of disability, community integration, health belief and refugee studies. His work in the last area has included research into the experiences of Mozambican refugees in Malawi and, more recently, analysis of the social integration of refugees in Scotland. He is a member of the Editorial Board of both *Health Education Research* and the *Journal of Refugee Studies*. He has worked with a number of agencies involved in refugee assistance, including UNHCR, MSF-Holland and Oxfam, with field experience across Southern Africa, South Asia, Eastern Europe and the Caribbean. The Centre for International Health Studies constitutes a lively, multi-disciplinary and multi-cultural environment, with staff, researchers and students drawn from Europe, South Asia, Sub-Saharan Africa and Latin America.

Daniel N. Berkow *UNCW Counselling Centre, Student Development Services,*
601–5 College Road, Wilmington, NC 28403-3297, USA

Daniel N. Berkow, PhD, is a psychologist who counsels students and teaches psychology at the University of North Carolina, Wilmington. His interests in research and publication are in the areas of intercultural exchange of ideas related to health and therapy, conceptualization of the self as this affects therapy, and uses of individual and group therapy to address awareness issues. He has a long-term interest and involvement in the study of the Eastern approaches to health and well-being embodied in Taoism, Buddhism, and Advaita Vedanta.

John Berry *Independent Consultant*

John Berry was formerly Professor of Psychology at Queen's University, Kingston, Canada, and is now engaged in independent consultancy work. He received his BA from Sir George Williams University (Montreal) in 1963, and his PhD from the University of Edinburgh in 1966. He has been a lecturer at the University of Sydney for three years, a Fellow of the Netherlands Institute for Advanced Study and a visiting Professor at the Universite de Nice and the Université de Genève. He is a past Secretary-General, past President, and Honorary Fellow of the International Association for Cross-Cultural Psychology. He is the author of over twenty books in the areas of cross-cultural, social, and cognitive psychology, and is particularly interested in the application of cross-cultural psychology to public policy and programmes in the areas of acculturation, multiculturalism, immigration, health, and education.

George D. Bishop *Department of Psychology and Social Work,*
University of Singapore, Singapore

George D. Bishop is a psychologist by training and teaches health psychology in the Department of Social Work and Psychology at the National University of Singapore. He is an Caucasian American citizen who is a Permanent Resident of Singapore and has lived there since 1991. His research interests include lay conceptions of physical illness, psychosocial factors in HIV/AIDS, and the role of emotion in cardiovascular disease.

Philip Cook *School of Child and Youth Care, University of Victoria,*
PO Box 1700, Victoria, BC, Canada

Philip Cook is Assistant Professor of Child and Youth Welfare at the University of Victoria, BC, Canada. He undertook his PhD at Queen's University, Ontario, in cross-cultural psychology. His research interests include human rights, indigenouos psychologies and health promotion in developing countries.

Adrian Furnham *Department of Psychology, University College London,*
Gower Street, London WC1E 6BT, UK

Adrian Furnham was educated at the London School of Economics where he obtained a distinction in an MSc Econ., and at Oxford University where he completed a doctorate (DPhil) in 1981. He has subsequently earned DSc (1991) and DLitt (1995) degrees. Previously a lecturer in psychology at Pembroke College, Oxford, he is now Professor of Psychology at University College London. He has lectured widely abroad and held scholarships and professorships at, among others, the University of New South Wales, the University of the West Indies and the University of Hong Kong. He has written over 400 scientific papers and 25 books including *Culture Shock* (1994), *The New Economic Mind* (1995), *Personality at Work* (1994), *The Myths of Management* (1996) and *The Psychology of Behaviour at Work* (1997). Professor Furnham is a Fellow of the British Psychological Society and is ranked the second most productive psychologist in the world since 1980. He is on the editorial board of a number of international journals, as well as the board of directors of the International Society for the Study of Individual Differences. He is also founder director of Applied Behavioural Research Associates

(ABRA), a psychological consultancy. He writes a regular column in the *Financial Times* and is a regular contributor to BBC radio and television. Like Noel Coward, he believes work is more fun than fun and considers himself to be a well-adjusted workaholic. He is, however, often sought after by bridge, tennis and squash players who like to win. He enjoys writing popular articles, travelling to exotic countries, consulting on real-life problems, and going to the theatre.

Pauline Ginnety   *Independent Consultant, Belfast, Northern Ireland*

Pauline Ginnety is a freelance researcher and trainer in the field of community health who has been involved in health promotion work in Northern Ireland for many years, and more recently in Bosnia and Herzegovina. She also worked as a full-time researcher and undertook anthropological fieldwork in Northern Ireland and in Zambia. Her Northern Ireland research includes work with Travellers, the Chinese and Vietnamese communities as well as local communities in Belfast and Derry. Her key interests relate to public participation in health and embrace folk health knowledge, inequalities in health, as well as the barriers experienced by some groups in accessing healthcare.

Daphne Keats   *Department of Psychology, University of Newcastle, University Drive, Callaghan, NSW 2308, Australia*

Daphne Keats is currently Conjoint Associate Professor in the Department of Psychology, University of Newcastle, Australia. She is a fifth-generation Australian of British background. She holds a PhD and MEd from the University of Queensland and a BA, Dip Ed. from the University of Sydney. She is a cross-cultural psychologist with a particular interest in Asian–Australian comparative studies. She has published books and many papers in this field based on research with collaborators in Malaysia, Thailand and The People's Republic of China. Since 1978 she has visited China on many occasions, working on joint research studies with colleagues at the Institute of Psychology, Chinese Academy of Sciences, Beijing. As well as working with Wang Shuguang on the general planning of his research, she spent a month in Chengdu when he was carring out his fieldwork, in order to become familiar with the locale and the work of the Chengdu colleagues who contributed so much to its support. In 1996 Professor Keats was honoured for her work in cross-cultural psychology by being made an Honorary Fellow of the International Association for Cross-Cultural Psychology.

Gillian Lewando-Hundt   *Department of Social Policy and Social Work, University of Warwick, Coventry CV4 7AL, UK.*

Gillian Lewando-Hundt has recently been appointed Professor of Social Sciences in Health at the Leicester-Warwick Medical School, having previously been Senior Lecturer in Medical Anthropology at the London School of Hygiene and Tropical Medicine. She was born in England, studied Social Anthropology and Sociology at the University of Edinburgh and subsequently was awarded an MPhil in Social Anthropology from the same university and a PhD in Sociology from the University of Warwick. She has undertaken field research in the Midlands of England and London, Gaza and the Negev. She is currently carrying out funded research in the UK, Kenya and Palestine. Her research interests are in the areas of social exclusion and health inequalities and the dynamics of gender, ethnicity and class on access to health and healthcare. She is also interested in the interface of anthropology and epidemiology and the links between research, policy and practice.

Anne MacFarlane   *Department of Primary Care and Population Sciences, Royal Free and UC Medical School, Rowland Hill Street, London NW3 2PF, UK*

Anne MacFarlane is a Research Fellow in the Department of Primary Care and Population Sciences, at the Royal Free and University College Medical School, London. Previously at the Centre for Health Promotion Studies, NUI, Galway, from 1992 to 1998, she completed an MA and PhD in Health Promotion. Her main research interests are pluralism and health-seeking behaviour, health services research and qualitative methodology.

Mesfin Mulatu   *National Institute of Mental Health, Bethesda, MD, USA*

Mesfin Mulatu is an Ethiopian currently on a visiting research fellowship at the National Institute of Mental Health, USA. He received his BA in psychology from Addis Ababa University, Addis Ababa, Ethiopia, and his MA and PhD in clinical psychology from Queen's University, Kingston, Canada. He is also currently a part-time student in the MPH programme at the George Washington University in Washington, DC, focusing on international health promotion. His research interests include exploring socio-cultural determinants of health and health behaviours, and cross-cultural issues in the assessment and treatment of mental illnesses.

Richard C. Page   *Department of Counseling and Human Development Service, 402 Aderhold, University of Georgia, Athens, GA 30602, USA*

Richard C. Page, PhD is a Professor in the Department of Counseling and Human Development Services at the University of Georgia. He has published over 80 refereed articles in professional journals and has written a book developing a theory of existential unstructured group therapy. He has had two Fulbright scholarships which have enabled him to teach and undertake research in the Department of Applied Psychology, University College Cork, Cork, Ireland. Dr Page is currently doing research in different countries on comparing the ways the self, feeling and counselling are perceived in these countries.

Karl Peltzer   *Department of Psychology, University of the North, Private Bag X1106, Sovenga, 0727, Republic of South Africa*

Karl Peltzer is a Professor of Psychology in the Department of Psychology at the University of the North in South Africa. He is also director of the Health

Behaviour Research Unit at the same University. His latest books are on *Psychology and Health in Africa* (1995) and *Counselling and Psychotherapy of Victims of Violence in Sociocultural Context* (1996), and his areas of interest are psychology and health in Africa.

Charles Vincent   *Department of Psychology, University College London, Gower Street, London WC1E 6BT, UK*

Charles Vincent is a British psychologist born in London in 1952. He is currently Reader in Psychology at University College London. He trained as a clinical psychologist working in the British National Health Service, and also trained and practised for some years as an acupuncurist. His PhD thesis concerned the treatment of migraine by acupuncture, but its central theme was the establishment of an effective methodology for the evaluation of acupuncture treatment generally. In 1986, with Phil Richardson, he published the first major reviews of the effectiveness of acupuncture as a treatment for pain. He has published extensively on the treatment of headache with acupuncture and on methodological issues on the evaluataion of acupuncture and complimentary medicine. Recent studies with Adrian Furnham have explored the psychological factors underlying the appeal of complementary medicine. His current research concerns the nature, causes and consequences of adverse events in medicine and the management of risk in medicine. He is Director of the Clinical Risk Unit at University College London which conducts research and provides training on risk management in health care.

Shuguang Wang   *Department of Psychology, University of Newcastle, University Drive, Callaghan, NSW 2308, Australia*

Shuguang Wang is of Chinese Han nationality, born in Chengdu, the capital city of the Sichuan province of China. His undergraduate and postgraduate studies were conducted at Sichuan University. From 1987 to 1993 he was Associate Professor and Director of the Sichuan Institute of Sociology. He has published seven academic monographs and more than eighty papers on China's politics, culture, education, social psychology and health-related issues. In 1993 he undertook further training in methodology for HIV-related research, incorporating a strong anthropological perspective, at South California College, USA. From 1995 to 1998, he was enrolled as a doctoral candidate in psychology at the University of Newcastle, Australia, where he successfully finished his PhD thesis on STD and HIV prevention in China.

Mee Lian Wong   *Department of Community, Occupational and Family Medicine, National University of Singapore, Singapore*

Mee Lian Wong is a public health physician by training and teaches public health, human resource management, and health education and promotion at the National University of Singapore. She is a Chinese Malaysian citizen who is a Permanent Resident of Singapore and has lived there since 1990.

Her research interests include health education and behavioural intervention programmes for STD/HIV control among sex workers, community participation in primary health care and health promotion for the elderly.

Marta Young   *School of Psychology, University of Ottawa, Canada*

Marta Young is an Assistant Professor in the School of Psychology at the University of Ottawa in Canada. She received her BA from Queen's University (Kingston) in 1984 and her PhD from the University of Western Ontario (London) in 1991. Born in England of a Canadian father and a French mother, she was brought up in various countries, including Guatemala, British Guyana, Colombia, France and Wales. Her clinical and research focus has centred on gaining a better understanding of the psychosocial adjustment of immigrants and refugees during resettlement. She has empirically studied Portuguese, Salvadoran, East Indian, Hong Kong Chinese, Somali and Haitian migrants to Canada. She is past chair of the International and Cross-Cultural Section of the Canadian Psychological Association and is currently Deputy Secretary General of the International Association for Cross-Cultural Psychology.

PREFACE

Although the interaction of health and culture and the ethos of health promotion have been areas of great interest in recent years, relatively little attention has been given to health promotion within the context of the multicultural societies in which most of us now live. With this in mind my original working title for this volume was *Promoting Health Across Cultures*. However, through the process of editing its chapters and giving myself the opportunity to reflect more on some of my own work in the area, I felt that such a title did not capture either their essence nor their ethos.

Somehow, the idea of 'promoting health across cultures' seems to imply that an 'agent' is doing something to a more passive subject—it is a 'being done to' sort of phrase. This book is about more than simply working across cultures, it is about working *with*, *within*, and above all, *through*, the psychosocial conduit of culture. I hope that the title *Cultivating Health* conveys these subtle but important points somewhat more successfully. In the first chapter I develop an argument which I believe justifies this different emphasis, and show how a philosophy of cultivating health applies as much to subcultures, contemporary multicultural contexts and future cultures as it may be taken to apply to the more traditional and encapsulated ideas of culture.

While emphasising that health can be cultivated through many different and varied social, economic and political contexts, I also hope that debates about the methods and meanings of psychology, sociology, medicine etc. can move beyond the fixation on a dichotomy of whether things are 'cultural or colonial' to whether things work, or not, within the particular contexts in which they are applied. I have described this notion—which I have referred to only briefly—as pragmatic vernacularism. This sort of empiricism can liberate debate stifled by an undue emphasis on the *origins of ideas*, rather than on the social, and in this case health-related, *value of ideas*.

In this book authors have been given more space to develop their ideas than is usually available to them in either journal articles or conventional edited book chapters. This has been to encourage them to deal with their topic in more depth and perhaps with greater reflection than they have otherwise be given the opportunity to do. In recruiting contributors I also encouraged co-authors (where appropriate) to reflect some gender, cultural, geographic or disciplinary variety between them. Where this has been possible I hope that the different perspectives bring into focus more clearly the richness and value of the data and theory presented.

While the majority of contributors to this volume are psychologists, our authors are also drawn from anthropology, medicine and sociology. More importantly, they reflect a variety of perspectives and approaches, ranging from in-depth single case studies of psychotherapy to large-scale interventions for HIV prevention, and more theoretically based model building. Surely such variety is necessary to grasp a topic as multifaceted as the one we are trying to tackle here. One common feature to each of the chapters is, however, that they begin with a brief case study. Case studies help us to identify with the people we are researching and/or intervening. Hopefully they bring to life what each chapter is about.

Many undergraduate and postgraduate students have shaped this book by their reading of, and commenting on, various chapters, and I am very grateful to them. Members of our Health Research Group have provided continued enthusiasm and bright ideas over the years, and I am relying on them to continue to do so! I am grateful to the editorial staff at Wiley for their patience and encouragement. Finally, to my family, and especially my two young and enthralling daughters, who have on countless occasions prevented me from disappearing to work on this book, I say *thank you*—I still have a life!

Chapter 1

Cultivating Health

Malcolm MacLachlan

PROMOTING HEALTH

For the last half century the World Health Organisation (WHO) has shaped much of the thinking on health and health promotion. In 1948 the WHO defined health as '. . . a complete state of physical, mental and social well-being and not merely the absence of disease or infirmity'. This definition of health, recognising that health is multidimensional and that it incorporates physical, mental and social aspects, reached beyond the previous rather simplistic notion that health was merely the absence of illness. The WHO's emphasis on a *complete state* of well-being is also now recognised as overly simplistic. Health is a relative term. We probably each experience health in some respects and are simultaneously unhealthy in other respects. For example, physically disabled people can lead active and healthy lives, making valued contributions to society (as long as society provides an environment that does not handicap them). At the same time, some of our very paragons of athletic vitality have been reported to suffer anorexia, depression and many other self-limiting disorders.

In 1986 the WHO produced a Charter for Health Promotion (The Ottawa Charter) which described five key areas of activity: building healthy public policy, creating supportive environments, strengthening community action, developing personal skills, and reorienting health services to primary and preventative health care. Many of the early successes of the health-promotion movement focused on the prevention, or risk reduction, of somatic diseases, including most notably the eradication of smallpox through immunisation and the real prospect of polio now being banished from humanity. Mental health promotion has been a relatively recent phenomenon.

Cultivating Health: Cultural Perspectives on Promoting Health. Edited by M. MacLachlan.
© 2001 John Wiley & Sons Ltd.

The field of mental illness has refocused its interest from psychogenics (causes), psychodiagnostics (classification) and psychotherapy (treatment), and become the field of *mental health*, where efforts to prevent mental disorder and enhance psychological well-being now flourish (Albee 1998). Furthermore, health promotion has sought to 'swim upstream' from the outflow of ailments requiring remedies to the source of these ailments, where people 'fall into the stream' of illness and distress.

In moving 'upstream' health promotion has not only located itself at the 'healthy' end of a illness–wellness continuum, it has also become less organically focused and has placed more emphasis on psychosocial, economic and political factors. Albee's (1988) formula, which encompasses most of the efforts in the prevention of mental disorder, summarises the major factors thus:

$$\text{Incidence} = \frac{\text{Organic factors} + \text{Stress} + \text{Exploitation}}{\text{Coping skills} + \text{Self Esteem} + \text{Social Support}}$$

The increasing 'socialisation' of health-promotion thinking has resulted in many acknowledging that health promotion is therefore to do with trying to get people to adhere to, or align themselves with, certain *values* regarding health. While it is certainly true that one can be overly relativistic regarding what defines 'health', it is also probably true that we often agree with what constitutes health and what constitutes illness. However, such agreement may hide a plethora of different concepts of health.

IMAGES OF HEALTH

Arnold and Breen (1998) provide nine 'images' of health, including health as the antithesis of disease, a balanced state, a growth phenomenon, a functional capacity, goodness of fit, wholeness, well-being, transcendence, and lastly, empowerment. Each of these 'images', Arnold and Breen argue, reflects a different frame of reference for health and these are reflected in different personal preferences, policies and programmes:

> 'The health care system, from the smallest unit of service to the entire system, reflects a particular image of health. . . . Each client's right to his/her own image of health must be guarded. . . . The health care professional does not override or negate the capacity of clients to form their own images of health.' (p. 12).

Arnold and Breen's (1998) categories reflect a panoply of views within multicultural North America. Yet one could add to these, or suggest other classifications, on the basis that every categorisation reflects a basic concept that is grounded in the life history of its beholder(s). Consequently, the very precepts of 'Western style' health promotion can be justly criticised when they are applied outside their context, for instance, in Africa (Airhihenbuwa

1995). Indeed, Seedhouse (1997) has argued that health promotion is *necessarily prejudiced* in that 'every plan and every project stems first from human values'.

Although some theories of health promotion acknowledge 'values' as being important, they tend to simply 'factor them in', as an additive variable, rather than acknowledging their central role in an individual's motivation to act within any particular social context. Thus while it may be argued that 'cognitive algebraic models' (Stainton-Rogers 1999) to some extent incorporate personal values, such values are not contextualised within the social and physical environment that give rise to them (see, for instance, the Health Belief Model; Becker 1986: Theory of Reasoned Action; Ajzen and Fishbein 1980: or Social Learning theories; Bandura 1986). In contrast, the Ecology Model (Moos 1979) is rooted in contextually constructed views of health and well-being. Here both characteristics of the physical environment (geography, architecture, technology) and the social environment (culture, economics and politics) are seen to interact with those of the individual (such as genetic heritage, psychological predispositions and behavioural patterns) to determine health (Gorin 1998).

LOCALISING HEALTH

'Community participation' has become the means by which to root health promotion in the lives of the people it is intended to enhance. Collaborative community action research (CCAR) adopts an ecological perspective wherein close collaboration between researchers, practitioners and citizens is fostered in order to achieve community development.

> 'This *resource* emphasis orientates researchers towards a setting's strengths, competencies and potential promise rather than its weakness, deficits and problems . . . A central component of CCAR is that action and understanding must be grounded in the understanding of specific ecologies and contexts.' (Weissberg and Greenberg 1998: 483–4)

It would now seem to be recognised that (1) health-promotion efforts are products of a particular (and therefore potentially prejudicial) view of health, and (2) the ways in which communities socially construct their well-being should be incorporated as a resource for health promotion. Yet a common theme underlying these two factors—*culture*—has not figured prominently in the health-promotion literature. Milburn has stated that:

> 'there is a need for a more flexible approach to theory building in health promotion. Principally, *the need to bring back culture* and the failure of existing theory to tap into the richness, complexity and diversity of human experience, argues for a theorising which will reveal those lay structures of thought and behaviour which are integral parts of every day health related behaviour.' (1996: 42, italics added)

CULTURE AS A CONDUIT FOR HEALTH

In many health-promotion programmes culture is seen as a barrier to their effectiveness. Mainstream programmes may be modified to take cultural peculiarities into account, to navigate a way around the cultural barriers to their effectiveness. This accords with a deficit model of culture, where cultural identity hinders behaviour change. However, another way of looking at cultural differences is as different conduits to health promotion. As such, cultural practices, norms, beliefs etc. become facilitators for, not barriers to, health promotion. While the content of custom and behaviour may vary greatly across cultures, cultures function to achieve solutions to life's goals (Helman 1994; MacLachlan 1997a,b). Effective health promotion embraces cultural complexity and recognises the necessity of identifying appropriate goals from within a cultural context, rather than simply modifying programmes developed from the context of a different culture. In reality all health promotion is grounded in cultural context (just as it is prejudiced because of particular values), but many who work with largely mono-cultural groups, or who focus on the majority culture, implicitly assume the 'normality' (and universality) of these cultural norms.

While much health-promotion work that has incorporated culture has done so from the perspectives of working *across* cultures, that is, with a cultural group different from the protagonists, more attention needs to be given to identifying potentially health-promoting cultural characteristics *within* groups. To illustrate this point we shall briefly consider drug abuse in Dublin, Ireland. The problem of inner-city drug use has been increasing at an alarming rate in Dublin since the early 1980s, but particularly so during the past decade (MacLachlan 1998). The Combat Poverty Agency has been active in attempting to highlight how the deprived social context in which people live often primes the conditions for high rates of drug misuse (Frazer 1996). The 'drug siege' mentality which has gripped many housing estates, along with parents' concern to prevent the (drug) abuse of their children, has caused a community-based response which has, at times, been quite remarkable.

Angry at the openness and intrusiveness of drug trading, residents started mounting patrols and building huts (from wooden pallets and sheet plastic) around their housing estates, so allowing them to keep a 24-hour watch on the activities of drug dealers and to report suspicious car registrations to the police, whom they considered only occasional visitors to their area. There followed regular marches against drugs, often cumulating in protests outside the houses of suspected drug dealers. It would seem that the majority of participants in these marches were ordinary citizens fired by fears for their children's future. Resident groups set up local treatment centres and then sought funding for them, contrasting with the sometimes poorly received initiatives of the local health authorities.

I have argued that such community reactions to the problem of illicit drug use should be seen not simply as a reactive, curative or even preventative response, but also as one which has the potential to be *actively health promoting* (MacLachlan 1998). Antonovsky (1996) has proposed the concept of a Sense of Coherence (SOC) as a central mechanism for promoting health. He argues that a SOC is created when people respond to a stressful situation by finding it *meaningful* (in the sense that they are motivated to cope with it), *comprehensible* (feeling that they understand the nature of the challenge confronting them) and *manageable* (believing that they have available the resources to cope with the situation). If a variety of problems can be responded to in a meaningful, comprehensible and manageable fashion, then a sense of coherence may be achieved and health-related benefits experienced.

Unfortunately many people inhabit environments that are demotivating, lack opportunities for fully appreciating the nature of many social problems and which are stripped of the necessary resources to manage life's problems. It is therefore in these very environments that community (re)actions, such as those described above, can themselves provide a vehicle for a sense of coherence. Responding to the threat of drugs in a manner which reflects a social meaning (threatened youth), a sense of comprehension (identifying the source of the problem to be social deprivation, inadequate policing, sparse treatment facilities and insufficient investment in drug-incompatible pro-social activities), along with fostering the belief that the problem can be managed (through the empowerment individual's experience as part of an active community force), are activities which are in themselves, health promoting. In this example of inner-city drug abuse, *health has been cultivated out of the context of social deprivation*. It has been a 'natural' and courageous response to the suffocation of local identity.

CULTURE, COMMUNITY AND HEALTH

The word 'community' originates from the idea of sharing a wall. By creating an enclosure, a wall also creates a psychological space that is common to those who share it—they share the responsibility for living in it. The ancients had the Forum as the focus (a word derived from forum) for their civic activities. The word 'focus' also relates to the idea of a 'fire at the centre', which could radiate both literal and spiritual heat. The ancients believed that places of such great social value were guarded by gods, for whom they would perform rituals in order to keep in good favour. By ensuring that only people who knew the correct etiquette were allowed to enter such places the ancients thus sought to cultivate a good relationship with their gods.

Such rituals and etiquette varied, distinguishing one community from another. Each community, enclosed by its literal or metaphorical wall, developed different customs. The word 'culture' refers to the idea of cultivating—as in cultivating a crop—a relationship, not only with gods but also with other members of the community. The health of individuals also related to the idea of cultivating relationships: if an individual's behaviour was somehow inappropriate, or out of balance with the needs of the community, then ill-health and suffering would follow. Intriguingly, the individual who was the cause of such imbalance was not necessarily the one to suffer; instead another person, or group of people, could suffer in their stead. Thus one man's infidelity could cause another man's sickness. In ancient times health was therefore a very public concern.

Many of these themes, of course, resonate with more contemporary cultures. Whether one considers 'Third World' rural communities, 'First World' inner-city communities, or the corporate identity of multinationals (such as IBM), the matrix of their daily interactions are cemented by common customs and relationships. People want to get on with each other. When harmony is disrupted by famine, the criminal underworld, stock market fluctuations, or whatever, relationships are strained, people are stressed and health is compromised. There are many psychological and physical benefits that derive from strong social support, high self-esteem, adequate coping resources and other aspects of a strong group, social or cultural identity (MacLachlan 1997a,b).

CULTIVATING HEALTH

In proposing the concept of *cultivating health* I am suggesting that we build into health-promotion programmes the ways in which cultures can create well-being for their participants. Here culture is simply a term used to describe how people knit together and how they distinguish themselves from others. Some of the cultures we may need to work with in this new century do not yet exist. They will be created by like-minded people seeking to achieve common ends and fulfil similar needs. Culture is not simply a tradition or artefact, with customs and etiquette from a by-gone age, to be resuscitated by cyclical needs to know our roots. Cultures, as guidelines for living life, will change as the context of our lives change. Health will best be promoted by taking into account how people live their lives.

Cultivating health is about 'growing' well-being. Sometimes such 'growth' will require a 'new' cultural identity, sometimes it can revamp an existing cultural identity, and sometimes it will require a 'working together' of ideas, attitudes and knowledge from different cultures. Cultivating health is about 'growing well-being' and as such is an appropriate term to describe the process of community participation and empowerment, especially when this works through the conduit of culture.

OVERVIEW OF CHAPTERS

Following this introductory chapter the book is divided into three parts. The first deals with the context in which health must be cultivated, and the four chapters within this part each contribute a different perspective. Mesfin Mulatu and John Berry begin by posing two crucial questions: First, 'how fundamental are cultural factors to understanding the domain of health and illness?' Second, '. . . how are we to approach health promotion and health care among ethnocultural groups living together in culturally plural (multi-cultural) societies?' Mulatu and Berry develop a taxonomy of different sorts of health phenomena (cognitive, affective, behavioural and social), bisected by a community and by an individual level of analysis. This is a very useful device for helping us to think through the interplay between multicultural-ism and health. Mulatu and Berry call for the integration of various extant models to provide a conception that is both comprehensive enough and flexible enough for use in multicultural contexts.

The third chapter by Gillian Lewando-Hundt examines 'good' reasons for 'bad' records. It is concerned with elucidating the factors that influence the information gathered to construct vital statistics; official records of birth and death, that punctuate our entry to and departure from this life. According to Lewando-Hundt, such information 'projects an image of people's lives which can form the basis of regional, national and international aid budgets and health planning'. It is therefore important not just to enumerate but to understand how social, political and cultural issues *figure in* the derivation of this data. This chapter examines the case of the one million Palestinians who live in the Gaza Strip, and in doing so makes visible the human meaning and construction—indeed distortion—of vital statistics. It is hard to over-emphasise the importance of this perspective; for if our very basic (vital) data can reflect many subjective realities, then cross-national or cross-cultural comparisons must be rooted in the social contexts from which they derive.

The fourth chapter, by Shuguang Wang and Daphne Keats, is a study of how the dual employment system in China influences the propensity to contract HIV/AIDS. Since 1982 China has had a dual employment system comprising the state employment system and the self-employment system, or *getihu*. By the end of the 1980s those in the *getihu* system had generally achieved relatively high incomes, economic independence and relative free-dom from the conventional lifestyle and attitudes encouraged by the state. Wang and Keats demonstrate how the different social contexts and sub-cultures created by the two employment systems—the conservative and moralistic state system versus the opportunistic risk-taking *getihu* system—contribute to the (greatly different) likelihood that members of each system will engage in HIV/AIDS risk-taking behaviour. This study demonstrates very clearly that health or illness are not just biological or even cultural events, they are also embedded within political, economic and a variety of social dimensions.

Philip Cook's chapter on 'Cultivating Health and the UN Convention on the Rights of the Child' concludes the first section concerned with the con-text of cultivating health. Cook argues for a 'rights-based approach' to chil-dren's health, moving beyond technology and disease responses to a more holistic perspective, including notions of family life, economic security, physical safety, community resources and civic vitality. The challenge for such a 'rights-based' approach to cultivating health is to apply universally high standards for child development and welfare, and to be sensitive to the values of different cultural traditions with their different expectations for and perspectives on children. Cook provides an insight into the complexities of how the aspirations of the United Nations are required to intermesh with national and community initiatives if the full potential of the Convention are to be realised.

The second part of the book deals with pluralism, that is, parallel approaches to cultivating health. In some cases these may complement and indeed enrich each other, while in other cases they may simply offer choice in the competitive environment of health care. While much has been made of how Western health care has influenced (or colonised) other parts of the world (see, for example, Carr, McAuliffe and MacLachlan 1998), the sixth chapter by Dan Berkow and Richard Page explores how Asian psychologies can be incorporated into the Western practice of psychotherapy. The major paradigms discussed, Taoism and Buddhism, are focused less on the notion of 'fixing' incongruous or inconsistent aspects of the self and more on finding harmony within the contradictions of life. The idea of being at peace with change challenges the Western notion of arriving at valued end states. Berkow and Page outline an approach to therapy that combines insight with compassion, and argue that 'Without compassion, awareness moves away from itself and becomes ignorance'.

The idea of complementary approaches to health-providing alternative perspectives on how we sense our selves—is also a theme running through Adrian Furnham and Charles Vincent's chapter on 'Cultivating Health through Complementary Medicine'. With well over a hundred different types of complementary therapy and diagnostic aids, Furnham and Vincent argue that for even the main types, their history, philosophy and methods of treatment are extremely diverse. Some of the more common themes relate to the ideas of an underlying energy or vital force; seeing the body as self-healing; seeing disease as symptomatic of underlying systemic problems; an emphasis on prevention and the attainment of positive health; and on the patient/client being an active participant in healing. While health can be cultivated through treatment of specific ailments, complementary medicine, (for instance, yoga or aromatherapy) also have great potential in their application to health promotion—you don't need to be sick to benefit from complementary medicine. Furnham and Vincent's thought-provoking review of the evidence for the effectiveness of complementary medicine challenges conservative Western sceptics to rethink the meaning of health intervention, process and outcome.

The third chapter concerned with pluralism, Anne MacFarlane and Pauline Ginnety's 'Boiled Nettles in May', explores medical pluralism in Ireland. This chapter considers health-seeking behaviours in the Travelling community in Northern Ireland, and the health-related folklore beliefs of children and 'seniors' in the Republic of Ireland. While the themes here resonate with the previous chapter, the emphasis is more on traditional indigenous alternatives to modern medicine, as opposed to the multicultural complementary approaches which are now popular in many Western contemporary urban settings. Bone setters and 'seventh sons of seventh sons' are among the traditional folk healers considered by McFarlane and Ginnety. The complementary medicines referred to by Furnham and Vincent have little currency among Irish Travellers, the less well off, or the elderly. This chapter nicely illustrates that pluralism, and our choices regarding pluralism, are embedded in a much broader social, political and economic context.

The third and final part of the book addresses three very different and quite specific perspectives on cultivating health: traditional healing in Africa; the well-being of refugees; and the prevention of HIV/AIDS in Singapore. Karl Peltzer's chapter on 'Traditional Mechanisms for Cultivating Health in Africa' provides a fascinating insight into how the social norms and lores of some African societies work so as to cultivate health and maintain social order. The array of problems for which 'Traditional Healers' are consulted is indeed diverse; including economic and occupational problems (such as unemployment or protection from jealous workmates after being promoted), family problems, sorcery and witchcraft, and security and legal problems (such as the protection of property). Peltzer reviews a number of indigenous methods ranging the lifespan, from enhancing community healing following death, to methods of family planning. He also discusses how such methods and their cultural and practical value should be incorporated into contemporary health-promotion programmes. The range and depth of Peltzer's experience of traditional healing has produced a chapter rich in the multivariate nuances of cultural meaning and health.

Chapter 10, by Alastair Ager and Marta Young, on 'Cultivating the Psychosocial Health of Refugees', argues for a 'holistic analysis of factors impacting adjustment, reflecting the unique cultural contexts and demands faced by each displaced person'. They consider the psychological effects of four phases of refugee experience: pre-flight, subsequent flight, temporary settlement or asylum seeking, and the resettlement or repatriation phases. Ager and Young argue for the increased use of psychosocial interventions, particularly those with an emphasis on community development. They also outline psychosocially appropriate forms of response in a variety of situations, from emergency situations to resettlement and repatriation. Trying to mesh sensitivity to individual's needs with the effectiveness of United Nations policy is a mammoth challenge which Ager and Young take us through with care and an awareness of the flux of cultural issues that form the corpus of many refugee experiences.

The final chapter in this book, by George Bishop and Mee Lian Wong, describes the authors' attempts to design sustainable interventions to prevent sexually transmitted diseases and HIV, in Singapore. Bishop and Wong concentrate on at-risk sex workers who are required to have monthly examinations for STDs. Discontinuation of their trade or even deportation result in discovery of HIV. This scheme, along with the underground nature of prostitution, undoubtedly prevent many complying with the screening. Incorporating the PRECEDE–PROCEED Framework, Bandura's Social

Learning theory and the Theory of Reasoned Action, Bishop and Wong describe an intervention to assist prostitutes with negotiating condom use. In only five months condom use increased, as did refusal of sex without a condom, and the rate of gonorrhoea fell. Bishop and Wong argue that the PRECEDE–PROCEED model is particularly useful for work with cultural and subcultural groups, since it lays out a systematic procedure for identifying interventions that are likely to be effective with the group in question.

THE PRAGMATIC VERNACULAR

Bishop and Wong's chapter provides an encouraging example of how a well-thought-out intervention can produce meaningful changes in people's lives. While some of this intervention built on principles of Western psychology, it also sought out the strengths of the context in which the intervention was needed. It represents a pragmatic matrix of pluralism.

In many parts of the world we have seen the rise of indigenous psychology as a fascinating and valuable study of 'local' psychologies, but also, at times, as a reaction against the apparent hegemony and insensitivity of Western psychology. Often it will not be possible to transpose Western psychological thought onto non-Western problems. Elsewhere we have considered how Western psychology may need to be 'reconstituted', 'restated', 'refuted' or 'realised', outside the context in which it was developed (see MacLachlan and Carr 1994).

Sometimes projects may need to proceed without a 'grand plan' and to inch forth in culturally acceptable incremental improvements (MacLachlan 1996). The Orangi Pilot Project is an example of how urban squalor in a squatter district of Karachi, Pakistan, can be overcome to produce positive social change, with very little help from either local or national government, or from foreign aid. The starting point for this project was the rejection of existing technical standards for sanitation as being too exacting and inappropriate to the local situation, and the adoption of piecemeal sanitation funded at the expense of local residents. Over 15 years the project installed 94 000 latrines, connected up to approximately 5000 underground lane sewers and 400 secondary drains. Significant improvements in health followed along with subsequent health care and literacy initiatives (see Pearce 1996; Carr, McAuliffe and MacLachlan 1998).

This is an example of what could be called pragmatic vernacularism (MacLachlan 1997b). *Pragmatic vernacularism* is about what works. Sometimes indigenous psychologies, ideas and materials will be such an inseparable part of the context that any dissolution of them, or any importation of an external perspective, will fail to achieve the desired ends. At other times, ideas, materials or methods from elsewhere may be needed to unstick a community from the context which prohibits their well-being. Post-modern vernacular architecture has shunned classical or symbolic forms, to craft instead what people actually like, what works for them. It is local, particular, not 'modern' or universal. Its concerns are about functionality, both psychological and physical. More importance is placed on *where ideas are going* than on *where they have come from*. We are now in an age when pluralism is necessary to cultivate health, both locally and internationally. We must move beyond the historic dead weight of concerns about national cultures and international colonialism, and embrace the pragmatic and the vernacular in our attempts to cultivate health.

REFERENCES

Airhihenbuwa, C.O. (1995) *Health and Culture: Beyond the Western Paradigm*. Thousand Oaks, CA: Sage.

Ajzen, I. and Fishbein, M. (1980) *Understanding Attitudes and Predicting Social Behaviour*. Englewood Cliffs, NJ: Prentice Hall.

Albee, G. (1998) (Ed.) Primary prevention of mental disorder and promotion of mental health. [Special Section] *Journal of Mental Health*, 7(5), 437–518.

Arnold, J and Breen, L.J. (1998) Images of health. In S.S. Gorin and J. Arnold, (Eds) *Health Promotion Handbook*. St Louis, MI: Mosby.

Bandura, A. (1986) *Social Foundations of Thoughts and Actions*. Englewood Cliffs, NJ: Prentice Hall.

Becker, M. (1986) The tyranny of health promotion. *Public Health Review*, 14, 15–23.

Carr, S.C., McAuliffe, E. and MacLachlan, M. (1998) *Psychology of Aid*. London: Routledge.

Frazer, H. (1996) *Submission to Government Ministerial Task Force on Measures to Reduce Demand for Drugs*. Dublin: Combat Poverty Agency.

Gorin, S.S. (1998) *Models of Health Promotion*. In S.S. Gorin and J. Arnold (Eds) *Health Promotion Handbook*. St Louis, MI: Mosby.

Helman, C.G. (1994). *Culture, Health, and Illness: An introduction for health professionals* (3rd edn.). Oxford: Butterworth-Heinemann.

MacLachlan, M. (1996) From sustainable change to incremental improvement: the psychology of community rehabilitation. In S.C. Carr and J.F. Schumaker (Eds) *Psychology and the Developing World*. Westport, CT: Greenwood Publishing Group.

MacLachlan, M. (1997a) *Culture and Health*. Chichester: Wiley.

MacLachlan, M. (1997b) *Psychology as pragmatic vernacular: beyond culture and colonialism*. Paper presented to Psychology Department, Univeristy of Cape Town, December 1997.

MacLachlan, M. (1998) Promoting health: thinking through context. In E. McAuliffe and L. Joyce (Eds) *A Healthier Future? Managing healthcare in Ireland*. Dublin: Institute of Public Administration.

MacLachlan, M. and Carr, S.C. (1994) Pathways to a psychology for development: reconstituting, restating, refuting, and realising. *Psychology and Developing Societies*, 6, 21–28.

MacLachlan, M., Chimombo, M. and Mpemba, N. (1996) AIDS education for youth through active learning: a school-based approach from Malawi. *International Journal of Educational Development*, 16, 1–10.

Milburn, K. (1996) The importance of lay theories for health promotion research and practice. *Health Promotion International*, 11, 41–46.

Moos, R.H. (1979) Social ecological perspectives on health. In G.C. Stone, F. Cohen and N.E. Adler (Eds) *Health Psychology: A Handbook*. San Francisco, CA: Jossey-Bass.

Pearce, F. (1996) Squatters take control. *New Scientist*, 1 June, 38–42.

Seedhouse, D. (1997) *Health Promotion: Philosophy, Prejudice and Practice*. Chichester: Wiley.

Stainton-Rogers, W. (1999) Keynote Address at Conference on Reconstructing Health Psychology. Newfoundland, 1–3 July.

Weissberg, R.P. and Greenberg, M.T. (1998) Prevention science and collaborative community action research: Combining the best from both perspectives. *Journal of Mental Health*, 7, 479–492.

Part I

THE CONTEXT AND CULTIVATION OF HEALTH

Chapter 2

Cultivating Health through Multiculturalism

Mesfin S. Mulatu and John W. Berry

CASE STUDY

CULTIVATING CHILD HEALTH THROUGH IMMUNIZATION IN SUB-SAHARAN AFRICA: THE NEGLECT OF CULTURAL AND CONTEXTUAL ISSUES

Children under the age of 18 constitute close to half of the population in many Sub-Saharan African countries (United Nations Children's Fund (UNICEF), 1999). Unfortunately, a significant proportion of these children die because of preventable epidemic diseases and many are left with chronic and disabling conditions that degrade the quality of their lives. Among several public health intervention efforts, immunization has been adopted fervently by public health institutions of those countries as an indispensable approach to the prevention of diseases and suffering. This has particularly been facilitated by the adoption of the Expanded Programme on Immunization (EPI) as part of the primary health services of these countries. The EPI has been collaboratively launched by the World Health Organization (WHO) and the UNICEF since 1974 with the aim of providing vaccine-based protection to children against six childhood diseases: tuberculosis, measles, polio, diphtheria, tetanus, and pertussis (Basch 1994; Murugasampillary 1994).

Although significant achievements have been recorded in improving immunization coverage in Sub-Saharan African countries, current reports show that only between 51% and 66% of the eligible children are fully immunized against the six diseases (UNICEF 1999). These coverage rates are significantly lower than the worldwide average rates of 80% or better. Thus, as many as half of Sub-Saharan African children are at risk of vaccine-preventable diseases either because they are only partially immunized or are not immunized at all. While several reasons are responsible for much lower rates of immunization coverage in Sub-Saharan Africa, including poor resources and grossly under-developed health infrastructure, the conspicuous neglect of socio-cultural and contextual factors in the immunization programs is believed to have played a critical role.

There are several cross-cultural issues that may be raised in the context of such health protection and promotion programs. One may ask at least two major questions: First, have socio-cultural factors with regard to immunization been investigated before immunization programs were implemented? Second, have Sub-Saharan African communities been involved in the design, imple-mentation, and evaluation of immunization programs? The answers to these questions are generally not affirmative. Immunization programs in Sub-Saharan African countries appear to have been designed, implemented, and evaluated without much regard to social, cultural, and other contextual factors (Murugasampillary 1994). The neglect of these factors may have affected the success of immunization programs in several ways.

First, it should be recognized that modern vaccination techniques, largely based on Western biomedical paradigms of health, are foreign to the people of the region. While the crucial role of vaccination in disease prevention is not questioned here, health planners must recognize the fact that its use without consideration of the local beliefs and practices has probably undermined its potential successes. To begin with, the idea of injecting 'medicine' to prevent illness is alien for many cultures. In reviews of the literature from African and other developing countries, Basch (1994) and Nitcher (1995) have identified several cross-cultural differences in the concepts of immunization. In some cultures, immunizations have been seen as generally ineffective or inappropri-ate to healthy babies or pregnant mothers. In others, immunizations have been avoided because they are believed to anger local gods or spirits. In yet others, immunizations have been seen as covert Western attempts to control fertility or to foster dependence on biomedical services. In general, poor coverage in immunization programs in Sub-Saharan Africa are partly accounted for by the absence of reliable ethnographic and epidemiological data in their design and/ or implementation.

Second, immunization programs require adherence to vaccination sched-ules and technologies that are less flexible and that neglect the social, cultural, and environmental contexts of the people for whom they are designed. Thus even where communities are convinced about the potential costs and benefits of immunization, contextual factors associated with vaccination technologies and schedules may deter participation in the programs. For instance, in many Sub-Saharan African societies there are strict rules and taboos with regard to the timing of outside contact with the newborn and his or her mother. The requirements that the mother and the newborn be present in health facilities, be seen by a health professional, or receive invasive inoculation procedures represent culturally unacceptable health practices in those societies where such taboos exist.

Third, multicultural issues within the Sub-Saharan African societies may also play a part in the poor coverage of immunization in children. Although often a neglected fact, it should be recognized that most societies in the region are composed of diverse groups of people. Owing to the fact that nations in the region are formed based simply on colonial convenience and on centuries of migration and relocation of people in the region, most countries are mosaics of several distinct languages, religions, and ethnic groups that have unique (and shared) beliefs and practices to restore, protect, or maintain health. Even though health protection and promotion programs designed for one cultural group may not necessarily be applicable to others, health programs in such societies have been based on the needs and the priorities of the dominant ethnic or cultural groups. Thus, the absence of a comprehensive adaptation of concepts, vaccination technologies and schedules to various cultures within each society has compromised the effectiveness of immunization programs in the region.

Finally, the national immunization policies and programs in developing countries in general, and those in Sub-Saharan Africa in particular, have been based more on predetermined policies and programs of richer donor countries and/or international agencies than on analyses of national epidemiological and ethnographic data (Murugasampillary 1994). These programs are often far removed from the realities of the Sub-Saharan African nations and remain unresponsive to the needs, priorities, and capabilities of the target populations. It has been suggested, for example, that the list of diseases for which EPI provides financial and technical assistance does not cover those vaccine-preventable diseases that are priority health problems in some countries (Murugasampillary 1994). In some cases, the sheer focus on meeting immunization coverage goals has fostered the perception of immunization as the only way of preventing childhood diseases and the neglect of other effective strategies including improving nutrition or sanitary practices (Murugasampillary 1994).

In general, immunization programs in Sub-Saharan Africa, despite notable success in improving child survival and quality of life, have significant room to improve in order to achieve the critical proportion of coverage necessary to curtail childhood epidemic diseases. Given that such programs take place in pluralistic societies, addressing multicultural issues in their design, implementation, and evaluation would be critical. Ethnographic and epidemiological studies would be initially critical to assess health-care beliefs, practices, and priorities of each community that will participate in the programs. Community members, opinion leaders, and local health professionals from each ethnocultural group should be able to participate in making the decisions regarding how immunization programs are carried out, monitored, and evaluated. It is only when such cultural and contextual factors are addressed along with improved vaccination technologies that immunization programs will achieve their potential health and subsequent socio-economic benefits to the populations of the region.

APPROACHES TO MULTICULTURALISM

In this chapter we begin by outlining some contrasting views on cultural diversity in general, both across and within nation states. Then we pose two questions related to health. First, how fundamental are cultural factors to understanding the domain of health and illness: are they superficial, allowing us to largely ignore their potential contribution; or conversely, is culture so much part of the meaning of health and illness that no understanding is possible without first taking the cultural context into account? Second, depending on one's orientation to the first question, how are we to approach health promotion and health care among ethnocultural groups living together in culturally plural (multicultural) societies? Should such groups be treated as minor variants (minorities) to a mainstream, and hence as side issues in a standard health system; or should they be treated as cultural communities, with their own cultures largely intact, and hence with their own health concepts, values and behaviors? The first is primarily a theoretical question, while the second is more a practical one.

In studying relationships between culture and behavior, three orientations can be discerned: *absolutism, relativism* and *universalism* (Berry *et al.* 1992). The *absolutist* position is one that assumes that human phenomena are basically the same (qualitatively) in all cultures: 'honesty' is 'honesty', and 'depression' is 'depression', no matter where one observes it. From the absolutist perspective, culture is thought to play little or no role in either the meaning or the display of human characteristics. Assessments of such characteristics are made using standard instruments (perhaps with linguistic translation) and interpretations are made easily, without alternative culturally based views taken into account.

In sharp contrast, the *relativist* approach is rooted in anthropology, and assumes that all human behavior is culturally patterned. It seeks to avoid ethnocentrism by trying to understand people 'on their own terms'. Explanations of human diversity are sought in the cultural context in which people have developed. Assessments are typically carried out employing the values and meanings that a cultural group gives to a phenomenon. Comparisons are judged to be problematic and ethnocentric, and are thus virtually never made.

A third perspective, one that lies somewhere between the two positions, is that of *universalism.* Here it is assumed that basic human characteristics are common to all members of the species (i.e. constituting a set of biological givens), and that culture influences the development and display of them (i.e. culture plays different variations on these underlying themes). Assessments are based on the presumed underlying process, but measures are developed in culturally meaningful versions. Comparisons are made cautiously, employing a wide variety of methodological principles and safeguards, and interpretations of similarities and differences are attempted that take alternative culturally based meanings into account.

Related to these three orientations (about how seriously to take culture generally) is the issue of how to deal with cultural diversity within plural societies. Diversity is a fact of life; whether it is the 'spice of life' or a significant irritant to people is probably the fundamental psychological, social, cultural and political issue of our times. As such, it affects how we think about health and deliver health services to diverse populations.

All contemporary societies are now culturally plural. There are no longer any societies that can claim to be homogeneous with respect to objective cultural markers (such as ethnic origin, language, religion), or subjective indicators (such as one's ethnic identity or personal expressions of one's culture). Such diversity elicits a variety of responses at a number of levels: national societies, institutions, and individuals can celebrate or deny it; they can share it or isolate it; they can accommodate it or attempt to squash it. Regardless of the attitude or course of action towards diversity, however, both history and contemporary experience provide compelling evidence that cultural pluralism is durable, even if its forms and expression evolve over time. Such continuing diversity challenges the conceptualization and functioning of all societies. It is likely that a long-established consensus about how to live together may no longer be widely shared, because so much of human behavior is demonstrably rooted in culture (Berry, Poortinga and Pandey 1997; Berry, Dasen and Saraswathi 1997; Berry, Segall and Kagitcibasi, 1997).

For many reasons (colonization, migration, enslavement) all contemporary societies have become culturally plural. That is, people of many cultural backgrounds have come to live together in a diverse society. In many cases they form cultural groups which are not equal in power (numerical, economic or political). These power differences have given rise to popular and social science terms such as 'mainstream', 'minority', 'ethnic group' etc. In this chapter, while recognizing these unequal influences, we employ the term *cultural group* to refer to all groups in plural society, and preface it with the terms *dominant* and *non-dominant* to refer to their relative power where such a difference exists and is relevant to the discussion. This is an attempt to avoid a host of political and social assumptions that have distorted much of the work on psychological acculturation and intercultural relations, in particular the assumption that 'minorities' are inevitably (or should be in the process of) becoming part of the 'mainstream' culture (Berry 1990). While this does take place in many plural societies, it does not always occur, and in some cases it is resisted by either or both the dominant and non-dominant cultural groups, resulting in continuing cultural diversity (UNESCO 1985).

There are two contrasting, usually implicit, models of cultural group relations in plural societies (see Figure 2.1). In one (the *mainstream-minority*), the view is that there is (or should be) one dominant society, on the margins of which are various minority groups; these groups typically remain there, unless they are 'gently polished and reclaimed for humanity' (as Montaigne phrased French colonial policy), and incorporated as indistinguishable components into the mainstream. In the other (the *multicultural*) view, there is a national social framework of institutions (the *larger society*) which accommodates the interests and needs of the numerous cultural groups, and which are fully incorporated as *cultural groups* into this national framework. Both implicit models refer to possible arrangements in plural societies: the

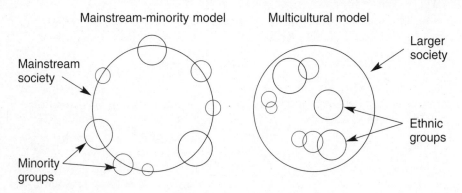

Figure 2.1   Cultural group relations in plural societies

mainstream-minority view is that cultural pluralism is a problem and should be reduced, even eliminated; the multicultural view is that cultural pluralism is a resource, and inclusiveness should be nurtured with supportive policies and programs.

Our answers to these two questions are explicitly pluralist. We consider that an understanding of culture is fundamental to understanding all behavior, including health and illness. With respect to the three orientations, we adopt a *universalist* perspective, viewing many aspects of health as pan-human in their roots and in their scope, while accepting that their definition, their recognition, their treatment and their care are all culturally rooted phenomena. With respect to the implicit models, we adopt the *multicultural* view, accepting that no program of prevention or care is likely to be helpful if the ethnocultural circumstances are ignored. In both cases, we assert that cultural ignorance is simply 'bad medicine'.

RELATIONSHIP BETWEEN CULTURE AND HEALTH

If these answers are valid, how can we proceed to engage in culturally sensitive health promotion across and within societies? One scheme (Berry 1997) is to recognize both the distinction (and the intimate relationships) between the cultural (community) and psychological (individual) levels of understanding. In Table 2.1 are four categories of health phenomena and two levels of analyses (community and individual). Crossing the two dimensions produces eight areas in which information can be sought during the study of links between culture and individual health. The community level of work typically involves ethnographic methods, and yields a general characterization of shared health concepts, values, practices and institutions in a society. The individual level of work involves the psychological study of a sample of individuals from the society, and yields information about individual differences (and similarities), which can lead to inferences about the psychological underpinnings of individual health beliefs, attitudes, behaviors, and relationships.

Table 2.1 Aspects of health phenomena considered at different levels of analysis

Levels of analysis	Categories of health phenomena			
	Cognitive	Affective	Behavioral	Social
Community (cultural)	Health concepts and definitions	Health norms and values	Health practices	Health roles and institutions
Individual (psychological)	Health knowledge and beliefs	Health attitudes	Health behaviors	Interpersonal relationships

The reason for taking cultural level health phenomena into account is so that the broad context for the development and display of individual health phenomena can be established; without an understanding of this background context, attempts to deal with individuals and their health problems may well be useless, even harmful. The reason for considering individual-level health phenomena is that not all persons in a cultural group hold the same beliefs or attitudes, nor do they engage in the same behaviors and relationships; without an understanding of their individual variations from the general community situation, harm may well, again, be inflicted.

Examples of work in the eight areas of interest are numerous in the research and professional literature. At the cultural level, the way in which a cultural group defines what is health and what is not can vary substantially from group to group. These collective *cognitive* phenomena include shared concepts, and categories, as well as definitions of health and disease. At the individual level, health beliefs and knowledge, while influenced by the cultural concepts, can also vary from person to person. Beliefs about what *causes* an illness or disability, or about how much *control* one has over it (both getting it and curing it) shows variation across individuals and cultures (Berry *et al*. 1994). For example, in one community, the general belief is that if pregnant women eat too much (or even 'normally'), there will be insufficient room for the fetus to develop; hence, undereating is common, and pre-natal malnutrition results, with an associated increase in infant disability. However, there are variations across individuals in this belief, with education, status and participation in public health programs making a difference.

With respect to *affective* phenomena, the value placed on health is known to vary from culture to culture and within cultures across sub-groups. Within cultures, for example, Judaic law prescribes that health is given by God, and it is the responsibility of the individual to sustain it; the value placed on good health is thus a shared belief among practicing Jews. However, there is significant variation in the acceptance of this value across three Jewish sub-groups: Orthodox Jews have the highest value, Reformed Jews have a lower value, and secular Jews have an even lower value on health (Dayan 1993). Also, within the three groups there are further variations according to a number of personal and demographic factors.

Health practices and *behaviors* also vary across cultures and individuals. For example, with respect to nutrition (Dasen and Super 1988), *what* is classified as suitable food and *who* can eat it are matters of cultural practice. Many high-protein 'foods' that are not placed in the food category in Western cultures (e.g. grubs, brains) are avoided, while in some other cultures they are an important part of the diet. Within these general cultural practices, however, individuals vary in what they can eat, depending on age, status or factors related to clan membership. The *social* organization of health activities into instructions and the allocation of roles (e.g. healer, patient) are also known to vary across cultures. In some cultures, religious or gender issues affect the role of healer (e.g. only those with certain spiritual qualities, or only males, may become a healer), while in others, the high cost of medical or other health professional training limits the roles to the wealthy. In some cultures, health services are widely available and fully integrated into the fabric of community life (e.g. Averasturi 1988) while in others, doctors and hospitals are remote, mysterious and alien to most of the population. In the former case, individual patient–healer relationships may be collegial, in which a partnership is established to regain health, while in the latter, the relationship is likely to be hierarchical, involving the use of authority and compliance.

APPROACHES TO MULTICULTURAL HEALTH PROMOTION

Although several definitions of health promotion are available, the WHO provides a comprehensive definition that is also useful in the context of pluralistic societies. It defines health promotion as 'social, educational, and political action that enhances public awareness of health, fosters healthy life styles and community action in support of health, and empowers people to exercise their rights and responsibilities in shaping their environments, systems and policies that are conducive to health and well-being' (Dhillon and Philip 1994: 9). By this definition, it is implied that health promotion at a population level can be achieved both directly and indirectly. Directly, health promotion may be aimed at health behaviors with appropriate cultural and other contextual issues taken into consideration. This may specifically involve changing particular life styles (e.g. increasing the frequency of physical exercise) through health education of individuals of diverse backgrounds. Indirectly, health promotion may target aspects of the larger social system so that positive health changes are accrued. In this case, the focuses of intervention are government health policies, organizational practices, and professional behaviors (Dhillon and Philip 1994; McKinlay 1993; Mechanic 1999). Improved national or international policies that promoted access to safe drinking water, comfortable working conditions, immunization services, sanitation facilities or adoption of healthy diet practices are some instances through which significant gains in health have been achieved in both developing and developed societies (Dhillon and Philips 1994; Mechanic 1999; Young 1998).

Health promotion programs in pluralistic societies appear to take one of the following approaches. First, cultural diversity issues may be completely ignored in the design and implementation of health promotion programs by solely focusing on the health care needs or priorities of the dominant cultural group, and hence embracing only the dominant health paradigm (usually Western biomedicine). This approach assumes, quite incorrectly, that health care needs, behaviors, cognitions, or resources are similar across cultures and/or they are immaterial in health promotion processes and outcomes (cf. the Absolutist approach).

Second, culturally informed programs focusing only on one 'minority' cultural group may be designed and implemented. For instance, in the United States, programs to promote physical exercise may be developed solely for African American, Asian American or Hispanic communities (cf. the Relativist approach). These programs may range from those with minimal cultural information incorporated (i.e. they are simply 'minorities') through to those with detailed ethnographic information and local community participation in the design and implementation of the programs. While this approach is a step ahead of the first one, it also suffers from failure to account for the dynamic interaction of health and culture among the diverse cultural groups and subgroups living in pluralistic societies.

The third approach to health promotion in pluralistic settings is multicultural in design and implementation. By definition, multicultural health promotion would make sure that all cultural groups are involved in health activities, decision making, and implementation of interventions. It would aim at making health promotion programs accessible and acceptable to diverse cultural groups by designing interventions that are sensitive to and informed about the groups' traditions, beliefs and practices (cf. the Universalist approach). Unlike the first two approaches, multicultural health promotion should mean moving beyond the planning of interventions for broader and ambiguous racial/ethnic referents ('minorities') such as Africans, Caucasians, Asians, or Hispanics. Even within the United States, both the majority and minority communities are far from being homogenous. For instance, the referent Hispanic in the United States refers to Spanish-speaking people including, among others, Mexicans, Cubans, and Puerto Ricans whose cultures and historical developments are quite different (Aspen Reference Group 1997; Lassiter 1995). Similarly, African Americans may be of several subcultures: the descendants of the former slaves that were directly brought to the United States, Caribbeans, or recent African immigrants (Betancourt and Lopez 1993). Similar cultural diversity is also found among European American populations (Lassiter 1995; Juliá 1995). In addition to providing culturally competent health education messages, multicultural health promotion efforts should also encompass the use of culturally appropriate methods of information dissemination, implementation monitoring, and impact evaluation. Effective multicultural health promotion, protection, or related intervention efforts should be flexible in selecting different strategies to accommodate the diverse needs, priorities, and resources of the cultural groups involved (Airhihenbuwa 1995; Aspen Reference Group 1997; Frankish, Lovato and Shannon 1999; Gardenswartz and Rowe 1998; Ramirez 1998).

CHALLENGES IN MULTICULTURAL HEALTH PROMOTION

The task of designing and implementing multicultural health promotion programs, briefly discussed below, is not an easy one. In fact, we can safely assume that some policy makers and health promotion planners may opt to ignore diversity issues partly because of the enormous time, effort, and cost it requires to accomplish this lofty goal given constrained human and mater- ial resources. This is particularly so in societies in which there are numerous distinct cultural groups (Buchanan 1997–8), including major metropolitan areas both in developed and developing countries. It should be noted, however, that overlooking or superficially treating cultural factors is much more costly in the long run than the initial costs incurred with appropriate multicultural health development. However, even when resources are avail- able, it may be difficult to achieve a truly multicultural intervention program because of long-standing and deep-rooted structural disparities and une- qual power relationships that exist among cultural groups. In this regard, one may argue that efforts aimed at reducing socioeconomic disparities and unequal power representation may qualify as crucial elements of multi- cultural health promotion.

Different cultural groups, by virtue of evolving in response to the de- mands of historically different environments, have different health prob- lems and priorities (MacLachlan 1997; Young 1998). Medical anthropologists and cross-cultural researchers also argue that culture operates both as a coping resource which members of the group utilize to deal with health- related problems and as a causative risk factor by directly exposing people to diseases and injuries (Hahn 1995; Helman 1994; MacLachlan 1997). Similarly, as we noted earlier, culture also defines what is considered healthy and how to maintain, protect, and promote health or well-being. While careful synthesis may make it possible to have a common ground for a health promotion program, variations in the distribution of health and disease, resources and barriers, health beliefs, cognitions, attitudes, and practices among diverse populations pose a serious challenge for health intervention planners.

Another important challenge in planning and executing multicultural health promotion may be in separating the health impacts of fundamental structural issues such as racism, poverty, or social status disparities from that of cultural diversity itself (Buchanan 1997–8). It is argued that these factors have a significant role to play in health and health intervention above and beyond cultural diversity, and that multiculturalism may be incorrectly used as a substitute for them, and as a result, distort the health effects of these structural issues (Buchanan 1997–8). The challenge here seems to be to finding a better conceptualization and measurement of multiculturalism, one that is independent of these social structural factors.

OPPORTUNITIES IN MULTICULTURAL HEALTH PROMOTION

One may ask why is there a need for a multicultural health promotion program? What unique opportunities would it create that would not exist otherwise? At least four broad benefits or advantages may be gained from designing and implementing health promotion that caters for culturally diverse groups in pluralistic societies. These parallel the general benefits of multiculturalism for a society as a whole (Berry 1991).

First, health promotion programs that are firmly grounded in cultural awareness and sensitivity, knowledge of sociocultural processes, and cross-cultural communication skills are likely to be more accurate and effective in reaching the intended goals among the diverse target groups than those which ignore the impacts of cultural diversity on health behaviors, cognitions, and outcomes (Kavanagh and Kennedy 1992; Jackson and Sellers 1996; Juliá 1995). This is a specific case of the general proposition that 'indigenous psychologies' are both more accurate and more useful than those imposed from outside (Kim and Berry 1993).

Second, successful multicultural health promotion would lead to the development of communal interest, a sense of interdependence and solidarity, and common destiny among diverse groups sharing a similar environment. This, in turn, would improve the social commitment to health and the sustainability of the programs even after the specific intervention is completed (Nilsen 1996; Ramirez 1998). Given that the success of health promotion efforts partly depends on availability and use of social support networks (Dhillon and Philips 1994; Mechanic 1999), multicultural interventions would make it natural for such networks to be strengthened and to be effectively utilized by diverse cultural groups.

Third, an often-missed opportunity in health promotion programs that ignore culture or diversity is the knowledge and practical skill contribution of minority cultural groups to health promotion, disease prevention, and clinical care. As we stated earlier, every culture has its own health concepts and health care system that are inherited from previous generations; each culture offers different and often effective pathways for healthy living (MacLachlan 1997; Juliá 1995). The synergism that can be created by having different and complementary approaches to the same goal is only possible under a multicultural health promotion context. For instance, efforts to improve cardiovascular fitness may be enhanced by adopting and incorporating non-Western health practices such as meditation and the avoidance of animal fat which partly characterize some Asian cultures.

Finally, given that health promotion programs, like other health care resources and services, are unevenly distributed among the diverse cultural
groups in pluralistic societies, multicultural health promotion offers the opportunity to partially redress the historically overlooked health problems
and priorities of the neglected (usually minority) cultural groups. In other
words, multicultural health promotion can be used as one vehicle by which
equity in health care resources would be attained. This concurs with the idea
that health promotion is a means with which people would be empowered
to exercise their rights and responsibilities (Dhillon and Philip 1994).

STRATEGIES FOR MULTICULTURAL HEALTH PROMOTION

There are three major target groups for health promotion programs in pluralistic societies: individuals, families, and neighborhoods or communities.
In addition, health promotion may be designed at the regional, national as
well as international levels for whole cultural groups, even though the effective targets or units of analysis largely remain individuals, families, or communities. Traditionally, such popular health intervention or planning
models as the Health Belief Model (Becker 1974), the Theory of Reasoned
Action (Fishbein and Ajzen 1975), the Stages of Change Model (Prochaska
and DiClemente 1983), and Social Learning Theory (Bandura 1986) primarily focus on individual-level factors including behaviors, cognitions, and
attitudes as their target of intervention. As a result, individual-level changes
have been the ultimate goals of health promotion programs. Recent health
promotion models, cognizant of the strong social and cultural basis of
health, give a crucial role to extended families, communities, and larger
socio-ecological systems (e.g. Airhihenbuwa 1995; Green and Kreuter 1999;
Ramirez 1998). Provided that health behaviors and cognitions are rooted
within the broader social context in which the person finds himself or herself, and given that these social contexts are different to members of different cultural groups, multicultural health interventions should pay
adequate consideration to familial and community factors both in their planning and implementation phases. In a North American or European setting,
for instance, health promotion programs involving immigrants from collecti-
vist societies are very likely to face serious obstacles if significant family
members are left out. At an international level, excluding native experts,
community leaders, and/or indigenous healers in the design, implementation or follow-up evaluation of any intervention would not only compromise the successful achievement of goals but also deny the target
community an opportunity for self-determination and pride in its own
cultural knowledge and practices.

Multicultural health promotion programs, like other community health
interventions, would follow at least a three-stage process of development
regardless of the intended target population or the theoretical models

chosen. These stages are (1) planning and designing the program, (2) implementing and monitoring the program, and (3) evaluating and refining the program (Green and Kreuter 1999; Kline 1999). Within each stage, several steps or tasks are involved and socio-cultural factors affect every aspect of the program development. We briefly describe cultural considerations that need to be taken into account in each stage of program development. Readers are referred to Kline (1999), Green and Kreuter (1999), and Bracht and Kingsbury (1990) for excellent and detailed coverage of socio-cultural and organizational processes in health promotion program development in multicultural or community contexts.

The stage of program planning and designing involves multiple steps and tasks including, among others, assessment of the needs and priorities of the community, developing appropriate tools and goals of intervention, and selecting health promotion activities that are suitable to the socio-cultural peculiarities of the target populations (Kline 1999). One crucial task in multicultural health promotion development is the identification of the health needs, resources, and priorities of each cultural group. Using one or a combination of needs assessment tools, including examination of disaggregated epidemiological data, focus group discussions with community members and local health providers, and/or conducting pilot surveys, it would be possible to isolate those health problems and health behaviors that are commonly perceived as a priority by participating cultural groups. Given the prevailing socio-ecological interdependence of diverse populations in pluralistic settings and the globalization of health problems (e.g. the spread of such diseases as acquired immune deficiency syndrome), finding such a target health problem or behavior would not be a problem. It must be stressed that culture-specific need assessments are essential to secure social acceptance of and commitment to the intended health intervention. Consider, for example, the case of promoting physical exercise across cultures. This is very likely to be an acceptable target in most societies but not necessarily perceived as important or a priority—as in the case of some war-torn Sub-Saharan African societies, where the predominant goal is survival. Thus, culture-specific needs assessment employing different approaches and involving the consultation of both health professionals and lay community members of each cultural group provides an accurate picture of the health needs that are perceived as a priority, the resources that are available, and the obstacles that exist.

Once the health priorities are identified, another crucial task in multicultural health promotion development is the socio-cultural analysis of the target communities or populations. Accurate understanding of the values, relevant beliefs and practices of each cultural group with respect to the health priorities identified would only be possible by conducting a thorough ethnographic analysis. This involves a broad understanding of all the phenomena noted at the upper (cultural) level of Table 2.1. Determining the health beliefs and practices of each cultural group may help identify culturally patterned *perceptions* that may facilitate or hinder individual, family, or community motivation to change (Airhihenbuwa 1995). Analysis of perceptions facilitates the recognition of the differences and similarities between the cultural groups in the target population as well as the possible actions that need to be taken regarding these perceptions during the health promotion program. Examination of community perceptions also assists in identifying strategies to promote perceptions that facilitate the targeted behavioral change and to resolve differences between promotion goals and contradictory health perceptions. For instance, in a recent sociological analysis regarding the rapid spread of human immunodeficiency virus (HIV) infection in Botswana, MacDonald (1996) noted several socio-cultural contributing factors including, among others, a strong social value for fertility and sexual virility. It is, therefore, imperative that health education programs against HIV infection address these cultural issues before assuming that knowledge about the pathogen or availability of protective methods would guarantee the adoption of safer sexual practices.

Ethnographic analysis would also help identify health behaviors and cognitions that Airhihenbuwa (1995) call *enablers* and *nurturers*. Whereas enablers refer to cultural, societal, systemic or structural factors that hinder or enhance change in health behaviors and/or cognitions, nurturers refer to the social networks (e.g. family, kin, friends, neighbors, communities) that would influence and mediate health beliefs, attitudes, and actions. Within multicultural societies, identification of systemic barriers to participation in health interventions for ethnocultural groups ('minorities') should be a precondition for health promotion efforts. For instance, various reports indicate that African American and Hispanic populations in the United States have lower access to health care resources and intervention programs (US Department of Health and Human Services (USDHHS) 1992; Giachello and Arrom 1996). Within the Sub-Saharan Africa context, health promotion or disease prevention programs that are costly, bureaucratic, and culturally and geographically distant are less likely to be utilized, thereby producing insignificant changes in health behaviors or cognitions.

The concept of nurturers appears to capture the importance of social factors in health that are often neglected in health promotion programs. Even when individuals are targeted, changes in health behaviors and/or cognitions are greatly affected by social network factors. Social networks influence the adoption of changes directly by providing instrumental or emotional support to the individual and indirectly by providing normative ideas about the appropriateness, importance, or effectiveness of the change. For instance, promoting fertility regulation in Ethiopia was significantly improved by involving both the husbands and the wives in a contraceptive health education program compared to other attempts that involved only the wives (Terefe and Larson 1993). This improvement is obviously the product of both the abatement of cultural barriers that render women less able to make family decisions and the improvement of social support available for women to initiate and maintain health-related changes. The values of social support networks as protective resources as well as facilitators of health promoting behavioral changes have been observed in other studies (Berkman 1995; Mechanic 1999).

Ethnographic analysis would also help identify the nature of salient behaviors and cognitions, their impacts on the health of members, and the potential approaches to deal with them during health promotion. Airhihenbuwa (1995) identifies three types of impacts: *positive* (i.e. behaviors/cognitions that have known beneficial effects on health), *existential* (i.e. behaviors/cognitions that have symbolic values to the cultural group but have no harm on health) or *negative* (i.e. behaviors/cognitions that are known to be harmful to health).

Every cultural group inherits from the preceding generations accumulated knowledge and practical skills that have been used to promote health and to treat or prevent illnesses. While most may be considered positive or existential, some may inadvertently expose individuals as well as the community to health risks. Multicultural health promotion efforts need to identify positive health behaviors and cognitions, and encourage their utilization, preservation, and maintenance as part of the planned intervention program (Airhihenbuwa 1995; Kavanagh and Kennedy 1992). Breastfeeding among Sub-Saharan African cultures, avoidance of alcohol among Muslims, vegetarian diet and meditation among some Asian societies are examples of positive health behaviors. Airhihenbuwa (1995) argues that these positive behaviors and cognitions are the 'culture's contributions to the global production of knowledge and meaning' and their affirmation by health educators not only empowers the participants but also makes the success and sustainability of the program possible (p. 33).

Some Middle Eastern and African cultures prescribe the wearing of amulets or protective charms to ward off evil spirits. This is an example of an existential behavior that is mostly harmless to health. Unless there is any reason to believe that these behaviors compromise the health of the individual, his or her family or the community, health promotion programs should not attempt to change them nor should failure of intervention programs be blamed on them (Airhihenbuwa 1995). They are better left intact because attempting to modify them without convincing reasons would likely lead to resentment from target populations and failure of well-intended programs.

Health beliefs and practices that are known to have harmful impacts on health such as withholding fluid from a victim of diarrhea, consumption of raw meat, avoidance of certain foods and female genital mutilation are practiced in various parts of Sub-Saharan Africa and elsewhere (Airhihenbuwa 1995; Dhillon and Philip 1994). Health promotion and protection programs should focus on modifying these behaviors so that their negative, sometimes fatal, health effects can be minimized or avoided altogether. In this case, it is suggested that careful understanding be reached about the perspectives of the members of the cultural group(s), and about the prevailing cultural, historical, and socio-political contexts in which these behaviors occur. More importantly, proposed changes should be made meaningful and acceptable to the community (Airhihenbuwa 1995; Kavanagh and Kennedy 1992).

Analyses of data gathered from both the needs assessment and ethnographic approaches should be able to provide a comprehensive array of information about the target health problem, its social-cultural and ecological determinants, the availability and accessibility of resources, and other potentially relevant factors for health promotion efforts. Analytical findings must inform the determination of the specific educational and programmatic goals and activities that would be incorporated into the program. In addition, the way these goals and objectives are to be achieved, monitored, and evaluated have to be clearly specified with the help of data and not be simply based on the planners' hunch. Ultimately, armed with ethnographic and epidemiological data, both health promotion planners and community members from the participating cultures must decide on the most appropriate intervention goals, objectives, and strategies to be adopted to address the health needs of each community. In sum, the stage of planning and designing health promotion programs in multicultural settings involves the identification of common health problems or needs through active involvement of the target cultural groups. Needs assessment approaches help identify the health needs, resources, and priorities of each cultural group. Ethnographic analysis provides a clearer understanding of the socio-cultural processes associated with the health problem or need identified. Collaboration between community members and health promotion planners assures that cultural differences are clarified and appropriate health promotion goals, objectives, intervention methods, and monitoring and evaluation approaches are chosen.

The second stage in multicultural health promotion program development is implementation and monitoring. This stage involves several activities that are directed at executing the health promotion programs formulated at the planning and designing stage. At least three interrelated tasks are subsumed under this stage: pre-implementation preparation, actual program implementation, and implementation administration and monitoring (Kline 1999). Pre-implementation preparations are those activities that need to be carried out before the program is initiated, including such activities as the identification, contact, development, and maintenance of support and sponsorship from community leaders, professionals, politicians, businesses, and administrators (Kline 1999). Community involvement and collaboration with stakeholders is a crucial pre-implementation preparation as it is for planning and designing the health promotion programs. Any program not supported by the power base of the communities it purports to serve is likely to be ineffective and/or short-lived. Given that different cultural groups have different resources and infrastructures, staffing needs, organizational structures, and resources available and needed have to be determined early before the program is implemented (Bracht and Kingsbury 1990; Kline 1999). Health promotion curriculum development, pre-testing, selecting and training program staff, and publicizing and recruiting participants are also very essential pre-implementation activities (Kline 1999).

Cultural competency training is fundamental in multicultural health promotion programs. Interventions in multicultural communities require that health planners are informed and sensitive about the cultural norms, roles, and beliefs of the target communities. In a similar way, Kline (1999) maintains that such cultural competency training may also be applicable to participants from the communities so that they would understand the professional culture (usually of Western biomedicine) of the health promotion planners. Beyond cultural competency training, the recruitment and training of participants from the target communities is recognized as a crucial component of health promotion programs particularly in pluralistic contexts. In addition to increasing the credibility of the program and allowing easier access to the target communities, the training of community participants helps develop new health leaders or promoters and paves the way for the sustainability of intervention efforts in the community (Aspen Reference Group 1997; Bracht and Kingsbury 1990).

Actual implementation entails that the target populations are aware of the program and that adequate resources are available to initiate it. In multicultural contexts, the publicity of the program needs special attention. Different cultural groups respond or have access to different types of messages or media. In addition to the usual written announcement of the program, multiple sources and mediums have to be used to reach as many eligible target populations as possible. Once the publicity of the program is confirmed, interventions can be applied all at once or gradually in a step by step manner among all target populations, or initially in the form of a pilot demonstration with only a small proportion of the target population (Kline 1999). Implementation efforts have to respond to prior and concurrent monitoring of the degree to which the program is being accomplished according to plans, policies, and regulations. Aspects of program implementation that require monitoring may include, among other things, timeliness of intervention activities, appropriateness of solutions to problems encountered, utilization and availability of resources, and preparation of oral and written reports (Kline 1999). As noted earlier, the appropriateness and acceptability of objectives and strategies have to be continuously monitored and modified to address the dynamic nature of health needs, resources, and cultural factors (Airhihenbuwa 1995; Aspen Reference Group 1997; Kline 1999). Meticulous monitoring should be able to help in program maintenance and consolidation by identifying achievements and failures early and suggesting appropriate actions.

Evaluation and refinement of the program represent the third stage in multicultural health promotion programs. While health promotion planners and administrators may have vested interests in the outcomes of the interventions, members of the target communities may equally deserve feedback about specific and overall effects of the program on the targeted health problems or behaviors. Thus, like in the preceding stages, the evaluation process should be a collaborative venture. Three levels or dimensions of evaluation are identified: impact, outcome, and process (Green and Kreuter 1999; Kline 1999). Impact evaluation refers to assessment of the program's immediate or short-term impacts. Examination of pre- and post-intervention changes in knowledge, attitudes, and practices associated with the target health problem represents an instance of impact evaluation. Outcome evaluation is another dimension of the evaluation process whereby the long-term social or health effects of the program are assessed usually after a lapse of a longer period of time. Objects of interest for outcome evaluation may include mortality, disease, disability rates, and other health status or quality-of-life indicators. Finally, process evaluation is considered when the intention of the evaluator is to assess the quality of the health promotion program elements, including the qualification of the staff, the appropriateness of the methods and strategies used, and/or the quality of participation of the target cultural groups in the activities. In addition to helping establish accountability of the planners, administrators, and other participants, evaluation efforts are essential to identify areas in which the health promotion program needs some changes, adjustments, or refinement (Kline 1999). While the intents and approaches of the evaluation of health promotion programs in pluralistic contexts may be similar to the evaluation of other community-level interventions, program planners should recognize that the timing as well as the dimensions of evaluation that are selected and used need to reflect the peculiarities of each culture involved.

PROSPECTS FOR MULTICULTURAL HEALTH PROMOTION

Increasing globalization of the market economy and migration of people are expected to create an even more diverse population worldwide. The health care demands of the world's population, despite diminishing resources, are also rapidly increasing. As a result, we would expect growing interest in and demand for multicultural health interventions, including health promotion. Issues of acceptability, effectiveness, and equity will also continue to be the driving forces of multicultural health interventions (Gorin 1998). Unfortunately, adequate models that combine social science concepts with public health are not yet available and are urgently needed. We believe that the integration of various theoretical approaches, including those that focus on ecological and socio-cultural processes (e.g. PEN-3 Model (Airhihenbuwa 1995); Eco-cultural Framework (Berry 1974)), those that target population-level factors (e.g. Health Canada 1994), and those that aim at individual behavioral and cognitive factors (e.g. Social Leaning Theory (Bandura 1986); Theory of Reasoned Action (Fishbein and Ajzen 1975)) would yield such models that are both comprehensive and flexible enough for use in various multicultural contexts. We also believe that it is only through the use of appropriate research and intervention paradigms founded on the commitment for social justice that the lofty goal of health for all will be achieved in multicultural societies.

ACKNOWLEDGEMENT

We are grateful to Rahel Adamu, MPH, and Cameron Norman, PhD, for their very helpful comments on an earlier version of this chapter.

REFERENCES

Airhihenbuwa, C.O. (1995) *Health and Culture: Beyond the Western paradigm.* Thousand Oaks, CA: Sage.

Aspen Reference Group (1997) *Community Health Education and Promotion: A guide to program design and evaluation.* Gaithersburg, MD: Aspen.

Averasturi, L. (1988) Psychosocial factors in health: The Cuban model. In P. Dasen, J.W. Berry and N. Sartorius (Eds) *Health and Cross-cultural Psychology: Towards applications.* London: Sage.

Bandura, A. (1986) *Social Foundations of Thought and Action.* Englewood Cliffs, NJ: Prentice Hall.

Basch, P.F. (1994) *Vaccines and World Health: Science, policy, and practice.* New York: Oxford University Press.

Becker, M.H. (1974) The health belief model and personal health behavior. *Health Education Monographs,* 2, 324–473.

Berkman, L.F. (1995) The role of social relations in health promotion. *Psychosomatic Medicine,* 57, 245–254.

Berry, J.W. (1976) *Human Ecology and Cognitive Style.* New York: Sage/ Halsted.

Berry, J.W. (1990) Psychology of acculturation. In R. Brislin (Ed.), *Applied Cross-cultural Psychology* (pp. 232–253). London: Sage.

Berry, J.W. (1991) Understanding and managing multiculturalism. *Journal of Psychology and Developing Societies,* 3, 17–49.

Berry, J.W. (1997) Cultural and ethnic factors in health. In A. Baum *et al.* (Eds) *Cambridge Handbook of Psychology, Health and Medicine* (pp. 98–103). Cambridge: Cambridge University Press.

Berry, J.W. *et al.* (1994) *Disability beliefs attitudes and behaviors across cultures.* Report from International Center for the Advancement of Community Based Rehabilitation. Kingston, ON: Queen's University.

Berry, J.W. Dasen, P.R. and Saraswathi, T.S. (Eds) (1997) *Handbook of Cross-cultural Psychology: Vol. 2 Basic Processes and Human Development.* Boston, MA: Allyn & Bacon.

Berry, J.W. Poortinga, Y.H. and Pandey, J. (Eds) (1997) *Handbook of Cross-cultural Psychology: Vol. 1 Theory and Methods.* Boston, MA: Allyn & Bacon.

Berry, J.W. Poortinga, Y.H., Segall, M.H. and Dasen, P.R. (1992) *Cross-cultural Psychology: Research and applications.* New York: Cambridge University Press.

Berry, J.W., Segall, M.H. and Kagitcibasi, C. (Eds) (1997) *Handbook of Cross-cultural Psychology: Vol. 3 Social Behavior and Application.* Boston, MA: Allyn & Bacon.

Betancourt, H. and Lopez, S. (1993) The study of culture, ethnicity and race in American psychology. *American Psychologist,* 48, 629–637.

Bracht, N. and Kingsbury, L. (1990) Community organization principles in health promotion: A five-stage model. In N. Bracht (Ed.) *Health Promotion at the Community Level* (pp. 66–88). Newbury Park, CA: Sage.

Buchanan, D.R. (1997–8) Editorial: Multiculturalism, racism and the training of public health professionals. *International Quarterly of Community Health Education*, 17, 213–219.

Dasen, P. and Super, C. (1988) The usefulness of a cross-cultural approach in studies of malnutrition and psychological development. In P. Dasen, J. W. Berry and N. Sartorius (Eds) *Health and Cross-cultural Psychology: Towards applications*. London: Sage.

Dayan, J. (1993) Health values, beliefs and behaviors of Orthodox, Reformed and Secular Jews. Kingston, ON: Queen's University Masters thesis.

Dhillon, H.S. and Philip, L. (1994) *Health Promotion and Community Action for Health in Developing Countries*. Geneva, Switzerland: World Health Organization.

Fishbein, M. and Ajzen, I. (1975) *Belief, Attitude, Intention, and Behavior: An introduction to theory and research*. Reading, MA: Addison-Wesley.

Frankish, C.J., Lovato, C.Y. and Shannon, W.J. (1999) Models, theories, and principles of health promotion with multicultural populations. In R.M. Huff and M.V. Kline (Eds) *Promoting Health in Multicultural Populations: A handbook to practitioners* (pp. 41–72). Thousand Oaks, CA: Sage.

Gardenswartz, L. and Rowe, A. (1998) *Managing Diversity in Health Care*. San Francisco, CA: Jossey-Bass.

Giachello, A.L. and Arrom, J.O. (1996) Health services access and utilization among adolescent minorities. In D.K. Wilson, J. R. Rodrigue and W.C. Taylor (Eds) *Health-promoting and Health Compromising Behaviors among Minority Adolescents* (pp. 303–319). Washington, DC: American Psychological Association.

Gorin, S.S. (1998) Future directions for health promotion. In S.S. Gorin and J. Arnold (Eds) *Health Promotion Handbook* (pp. 401–420). St Louis, MI: Mosby.

Green, L.W. and Kreuter, M.W. (1999) *Health Promotion Planning: An educational and ecological approach* (3rd edn). Mountain View, CA: Mayfield.

Hahn, R.A. (1995) *Sickness and Healing: An anthropological perspective*. New Haven, CT: Yale University Press.

Health Canada (1994) *Strategies for Population Health: Investing in health of Canadians*. Ottawa, Canada: author.

Helman, C.G. (1994) *Culture, Health, and Illness: An introduction for health professionals* (3rd edn). Oxford: Butterworth-Heinemann.

Howe-Murphy, R., Ross, H., Tseng, R. and Hartwig, R. (1989) Effecting change in multicultural health promotion: A systems approach. *Journal of Allied Health*, 18, 291–305.

Jackson, J. and Sellers, S.L. (1996) Psychological, social, and cultural perspectives on minority health in adolescence: A life-course framework. In D.K. Wilson, J.R. Rodrigue and W.C. Taylor (Eds) *Health-promoting and Health Compromising Behaviors among Minority Adolescents* (pp. 29–49). Washington, DC: American Psychological Association.

Juliá, M.C. (1996) *Multicultural Awareness in the Health Care Professions*. Boston, MA: Allyn & Bacon.

Kavanagh, K.H. and Kennedy, P.H. (1992) *Promoting Cultural Diversity: Strategies for health care professionals.* Newbury Park, CA: Sage.

Kim, U. and Berry, J.W. (Eds) (1993) *Indigenous Psychologies.* London: Sage.

Kline, M.V. (1999) Planning health promotion and disease prevention programs in multicultural populations. In R.M. Huff and M.V. Kline (Eds) *Promoting Health in Multicultural Populations: A handbook for practitioners* (pp. 73–102). Thousand Oaks, CA: Sage.

Kreps, G.L. and Kunimoto, E.N. (1994) *Effective Communication in Multicultural Health Care Settings.* Thousand Oaks, CA: Sage.

Lassiter, S.M. (1995) *Multicultural Clients: A professional handbook for health care providers and social workers.* Westport, CN: Greenwood.

MacDonald, D.S. (1996) Notes on the socio-economic and cultural factors influencing the transmission of HIV in Botswana. *Social Science and Medicine,* 42, 1325–1333.

MacLachlan, M. (1997) *Culture and Health.* Chichester: Wiley.

McKinlay, J.B. (1993) The promotion of health through planned sociopolitical change: Challenges for research and policy. *Social Science and Medicine,* 36, 109–117.

Mechanic, D. (1999) Issues in promoting health. *Social Science and Medicine,* 48, 711–718.

Murugasampillay, S. (1996) Who determines national health policies? In F.T. Cutts and P.G. Smith (Eds) *Vaccination and World Health* (pp. 195–211). Chichester: Wiley.

Nichter, M. (1995) Vaccinations in the Third World: A consideration of community demand. *Social Science and Medicine,* 41, 617–632.

Nilsen, Ø. (1996) Community health promotion: Concepts and lessons from contemporary sociology. *Health Policy,* 36, 167–183.

Prochaska, J.O. and DiClemete, C.C. (1983) Stages and processes of self-change of smoking: Toward an integrated model of change. *Journal of Consulting and Clinical Psychology,* 51, 390.

Ramirez, M. (1997) *Multicultural/multiracial Psychology.* Northvale, NJ: Aronson.

Terefe, A. and Larson, C.P. (1993) Modern contraception use in Ethiopia: Does involving husbands make a difference? *American Journal of Public Health,* 83, 1567–1571.

United States Department of Health and Human Services (1992) *Healthy People 2000: National health promotion and disease prevention objectives.* Boston, MA: Jones & Bartlett.

Williams, C. and Berry, J.W. (1991) Primary prevention of acculturative stress among refugees. *American Psychologists,* 46, 632–641.

Young, T.K. (1998) *Population Health: Concepts and methods.* New York: Oxford University Press.

United Nations Children's Fund (1999) *The State of the World's Children 1999.* New York: author.

Chapter 3

'Good' Reasons for 'Bad' Records: The Social, Political and Cultural Context of Vital Registration

Gillian Lewando-Hundt

'The Palestinian predicament: finding an 'official place for yourself in a system that makes no allowances for you, which means endlessly improvising solutions for the problem of finding a missing loved one, of planning a trip, of entering a school, on whatever bit of paper is at hand. Constructed and deconstructed, ephemera are what we negotiate with, since we authorize no part of the world and only influence increasingly small bits of it. In any case, we keep going.' (Said 1986: 37)

Vital statistics which make up vital registrations are records of birth and death which mark the beginning and end of life. They are vital to the individual, the family and the nation/state and have a multitude of functions and meanings. This chapter will discuss the social, political and cultural context of vital statistics. It will argue that consideration of the cultural validity and social meaning of vital statistics is critical in order to improve vital registration. The collection and analysis of the statistics needs to be underpinned by an understanding of their meaning. This may require qualitative research to explore the way in which data is collected, the perceptions of birth, death and marriage that people hold and the process they undergo to register these events.

According to May: 'there are three schools of thought on official statistics. First, the realist school of thought, second, the institutionalist school of

Cultivating Health: Cultural Perspectives on Promoting Health. Edited by M. MacLachlan.
© 2001 John Wiley & Sons Ltd.

thought and finally the radical school of thought.' (1993: 57) The realist approach perceives official statistics as objective measurements of real phenomena. The institutionalist approach does not perceive official statistics as objective and reviews the statistics in the context of the organisation which collects them in terms of its objectives and processes. The radical approach is similar to the institutionalist in being interested in the organisational context but also relates the official statistics to wider aspects of the dynamics and structure of the society within which they are collected. This chapter is written using the institutionalist and radical schools of thought in its approach to looking at the process of birth registration in Gaza in 1995–1997.

The first part of this chapter presents the case study concerning birth registration which arose unexpectedly during data collection in a research study in Gaza in 1995. The case study presented here is a shortened version of a published paper. The wider implications of the subject will be explored in the second part of the chapter.

CASE STUDY

BIRTH REGISTRATION IN GAZA IN 1995–1997
(based on Lewando-Hundt *et al.* 1999)

Specific Setting

Approximately 1 million Palestinians live in the Gaza Strip under the government of the Palestinian National Authority. The Gaza Strip is a narrow band of land wedged between the Mediterranean Sea and Israel. Palestinians in Gaza are either residents whose families have lived in the area for centuries or are descended from refugees who entered Gaza in or shortly after 1948. Approximately 75–80% of the population are descended from refugees who entered the Gaza Strip during the Arab–Israeli conflict of 1948.

From the early 1950s, the Gaza Strip was controlled by Egypt. Its inhabitants were not given Egyptian citizenship but were given travel documents issued by Egypt. In 1967, Israel occupied the Gaza Strip. From December 1987–1994, there was a popular uprising (*intifada*) which resulted in the peace process inaugurated by the Oslo Accords and which led to the establishment of the Palestinian National Authority in 1994.

At this time, the Palestinian Ministry of Health (MoH) took over the health services that had previously been administered by the Israeli Civil Administration. These consisted of primary health-care clinics and hospitals including all registration systems which were based on identity card numbers (IDs) allocated at birth. Within the last three years, the Ministry of Health has expanded the services based on a National Health Plan and there has been considerable investment in human resources and the development of the health-care system.

The health services today are provided by the Ministry of Health (MoH of the Palestinian Authority (PNA)), the United Nations Relief and Works Agency

(UNRWA), non-governmental organisations (NGOs), and the private sector. The UNRWA health services are mainly primary health care in the community and are provided free of charge to those registered as refugees. The Ministry of Health services are provided free to pregnant women and children under the age of 3 years. Other Ministry of Health services such as hospitalisation for childbirth or curative in and outpatient care are available to the 53% of Gazans who have health insurance. (Health Research and Planning Directorate, MoH 1997; UNRWA Annual Report 1996; UNDP 1996; Proceedings of the Technical Workshop 1994; Schnitzer and Roy 1994).

An example of the multiple provision is health care for deliveries. There are six UNRWA maternities with 60 beds and there are three MoH maternities with 24 beds attended by midwives. These provide free delivery services. In addition, 40% of all deliveries occur in government hospitals where non-insured families are charged US$40. There are also home deliveries attended by birth attendants or relatives (10%), private clinics directed by local obstetricians and NGOs also have three private hospitals which take deliveries.

The population of the Gaza Strip is characterised by a high birth rate (40.1/1000 in 1996) and in the same year the total fertility rate was estimated to be 6 births per woman compared to 7.4 births per woman in 1993. Infant mortality is relatively low and is estimated to be 25 per 1000. This is due to good access to health services, near-total coverage of immunizations, and control activities for gastro-intestinal and respiratory diseases (MoH 1996). There has been a marked increase in the population in addition to natural growth, owing to returning Palestinians who have settled in the area since 1994.

The data presented here derive from an evaluation and intervention study of maternal and child health services (MCH) to Palestinians in Gaza, funded by the European Commission DGXII Avicenne Initiative. The study aimed to evaluate and improve Maternal and Child Health Care (MCH) to Palestinians in Gaza using research which combined, conceptually and methodologically, anthropology and epidemiology (Lewando-Hundt 1996). The study covered three areas of the Gaza Strip.

(1) The Rimal district of Gaza City has a mixed population of residents and refugees totaling about 60 000 people (Abed 1992). It is the most developed part of Gaza and the area is characterised by modern buildings with satisfactory water and sewage services. Curative health services are provided by governmental and non-governmental organisations, refugees attending the UNRWA clinic or any of the others.

(2) Jabalia village with an economy which was once based on growing fruit and vegetables is situated three kilometres to the north of Gaza City. As farm land has been developed to provide housing for the rapidly growing urban population, the agricultural sector has declined and people have been forced to seek employment elsewhere. The vast majority of the population of 24 000 (Abed 1992) are residents of Gaza and are not registered as refugees. There is an MoH clinic as well as private practitioners.

(3)   Jabalia Camp, adjacent to Jabalia village with a population of 79 000, is
       the largest and most densely populated refugee camp in Gaza. It has an
       UNRWA health centre. UNRWA also runs the schools in the camp and
       other facilities in the camp. The housing resembles that in crowded periur-
       ban shanty towns. It was originally a temporary camp of tents for refugees
       from southern Palestine (now southern Israel) in 1948 which has become
       permanent with the tents being replaced by poor-quality crowded housing
       with running water, sewage and electricity.

Sample and MIS System

As part of the first stage of evaluation, 600 home interviews with mothers of
2-month-old babies were planned in these three neighbourhoods. Since the
infants had to be 2 months old at the time of interview, births of August,
September and October were selected for interview in October, November and
December respectively.

The birth information was selected from the management information system
(MIS) records kept by the Gaza Health Services Research Centre of the Ministry
of Health, Palestinian National Authority. This system records all births and
deaths in the Gaza Strip. The information is entered on a database from birth
and death certificates. It is a population-based system which has the following
information entered—identity card number of the baby and father, name, address including house number and street, date of birth, place of birth and
telephone number.

Each birth certificate has an identity card number allocated at birth. When
the child reaches 16 years of age, he or she will be issued with an identity card
with this number by the Palestinian Ministry of the Interior. This is a system
which was instituted by the Israeli Civil Administration in 1969 after a census
of the Gaza population. The same system operates in Israel. Identity cards are
used by both authorities to identify people. When crossing the border to Israel,
every Palestinian needs to have their ID card and a magnetic card with permission to enter. Without an ID card, entry is not possible. Hence the ID numbers
issued with birth certificates are a vital part of administrative control of the
population.

Unexpectedly, the interviewers had difficulty in locating the mother–infant
pairs on the basis of the information obtained from the MIS system. Many of the
addresses were incomplete. The interviewers developed a number of additional strategies to locate the families. Checking the clinic health records was
ineffective as addresses were similarly incomplete; making phone calls to
people with the same family name was also of limited use as few people had
telephones. The most effective strategy was to work with a local clinic nurse
and driver who were well known in the neighbourhoods and finally 450 out of
600 mothers were located.

As a result of these difficulties, it was decided to check the accuracy and
validity of the information for the sample of mothers being visited in October
(i.e. August births, see Table 3.1). These data, in particular the 100%

Table 3.1   Accuracy of 142 births registered in August 1996 as checked by home interviews with the mothers in October 1996

Type of information	Correct	(%)	Correct	(%)
Locality	137	(96.5)	5	(3.5)
Family name	114	(80.3)	28	(19.7)
Date of birth	139	(97.9)	3	(2.1)
Place of birth	128	(90.1)	14	(9.9)
Address	0	(0)	142	(100)

incompleteness of addresses caused some concern when discussed with the research team. The records of these August births from the data base were reanalysed in more detail.

Addresses

Reanalysis of the 206 addresses revealed that 127 (61.7%) records listed only the house number without the street name, 17 (8.3%) were incorrect in terms of having the wrong locality and address, and 62 (30.1%) were completely non-indicative. In summary, whereas the information was accurate concerning the locality and the date of birth it was less accurate concerning the place of birth and 100% of the addresses given were incomplete.

The team and members of the Research Centre came up with a number of explanations of these findings:

(1)   The population was more mobile within the Gaza Strip than was previously realised. People move but do not change the address on their ID cards and then when the baby is born, they register the baby at the same address as the father even though it is a wrong address. Ministry of Interior regulations were that birth certificates are invalid if the baby has a different address from the father.

(2)   At that time of political transition there were few street names or house numbers in the Gaza Strip. They were taken down during the *intifada* and had only recently started being put up again. One team member said that she tripped over the house number and street name of her in-laws' house whenever she hung up the laundry to dry on their roof in one of the refugee camps.

(3)   The Israel Civil Administration stressed the importance of ID numbers when putting together the MIS system for this was what was relevant to border control for the issuing of permits to work in Israel. Addresses were less important and never therefore stressed.

Despite careful database maintenance and inputting, it was clear how many babies were being born and when they were being born, but it was unclear where they lived. It was decided to trace the pathway of information from parents to the birth certificate in order to understand how inaccuracies arose and gain a clear idea of how to implement an intervention to improve the MIS system. Field visits were undertaken to the hospital discharge office, the hospital obstetric ward, offices of clerks, some clinics with birthing rooms and the Ministry of Interior.

Field Visits

There was no standard form for notification of a birth at the time of the field visits in early 1996. The hospital had a discharge form, UNRWA and government clinics had different forms and private clinic doctors gave out handwritten letters. If the child was born in the hospital, the parents would bring a discharge form from the ward to the hospital discharge office. From there, they would take the stamped form to the clerk (*Kaatib*) in a small office across the street who typed out a birth certificate application based on the information on the hospital form.

The clerk had to fill in the address which was on the father's ID card. If the address for the child is different from the one for the father, the birth certificate application is rejected by the Ministry of the Interior. Births which occurred in the clinics rather than the hospital were often typed up near the Ministry of the Interior. They also reported filling in the address of the father's ID regardless of actual residence. Next the typed forms were taken by the parents back to the delivery agency to be stamped and were then taken to the Palestinian Ministry of the Interior where four copies of the birth certificate were made: one stayed with the Ministry, one went to the Israeli Civil Administration, one went for entry in the MIS system at the Gaza Health Services Research Centre and a final birth certificate was sent to the relevant municipality who sent them on to the families. This process took from two weeks to a month.

Observation during the field visits revealed an additional problem: sometimes the birthweight was missing on the hospital discharge forms. The clerk next to the hospital said that he generally typed in 3 kg. when there was no information. (This hospital has 40% of the births in Gaza and most of the high-risk deliveries so that the proportion of low-birthweight births is possibly higher at the hospital than in the other settings). A hospital obstetrician's comments on the birth registration system were trenchant: 'Its all lies: there is no system.'

He added that if he wanted to carry out research on low birthweight, he could not possibly use the MIS data from the birth certificates for the data misrepresented the health of the Palestinian people. The obstetricians said that they themselves should not be involved in the process of filling in information for birth certificates. They added that owing to their busy medical workload, they checked only a few details such as name, ID number and sex, that the current system is 'a nonsense' and that they have lost the sense of importance of some information such as the weight of the baby. The hospital obstetricians fully supported overhauling the current system and wanted the doctor's signature removed from the birth certificate application form. Clerks based near the Ministry of the Interior reported that if birthweight was missing, they would leave it blank. They said that they also occasionally received birth notification without any stamp of a delivery agency.

Interventions

Two interventions were developed on the basis of the discoveries of the field-work, one concerning addresses and the other the birthweight.

Addresses

A meeting was held with representatives from the Ministry of the Interior and the Ministry of Health in order to develop a new system of birth registration. A new form was designed with spaces for the address of the father as indicated on his ID card and the 'real' address of the family. This would be a standard form used by all agencies, would have serial numbers and would be in triplicate so that a copy could remain at the place of delivery. Clerks would only be able to fill in a birth registration form when presented with this standard stamped form.

This system was launched in January 1997 with advertisements on the Palestinian Broadcasting Corporation television station. After a trial period of six months, the form was withdrawn for revision owing to complaints from the different agencies about the form's complexity and there has been no improvement in the recording of complete addresses.

Birthweight

The second intervention focused on improving the accuracy of birthweight recording. Since 43% of the births were taking place in the government hospital the doctors and clerk of this hospital were the starting point. A review of statistics from various sources on the first quarter of 1997 has established that there is a marked improvement in the accurate recording of birthweight on the birth notification form that the clerk in his office near the hospital fills out.

Tables 3.2 and 3.3 present the birthweight of live births in the Shifa hospital in the first quarter of 1996 and 1997 respectively. In 1996 3.1% of births were below 2500 g. In 1997 7.1% of births were below 2500 g. There still remains a discrepancy between the birth notification forms as filled in by the clerk and the hospital discharge forms filled in the physicians.

Data on the first quarter of 1997 based on hospital discharge forms are shown in Table 3.4. The total low birthweight at the hospital according to this source is 9.1%. This indicates that there is still many a slip between cup and lip in the journey from the ward through the hospital discharge office to the clerk over the road.

Although the underecording of low birthweight has been partially rectified at Shifa hospital through working with the doctors, discharge clerks and neighbourhood clerk, there remains a problem of underecording in the practice of doctors and clerks in other areas of the Gaza Strip. This is evident from the figures for the whole of the Gaza Strip for the first quarter of 1997 which has births below 2500 g at 3.5% (0.7% <1500 gms and 2.8% between 1500–2499 g) (MIS Unit, Gaza Health Services Research Centre, MoH, PNA). Further work

Table 3.2 Live births in Shifa hospital: deliveries by birthweight. (January–March 1996: data from birth notifications)

Age of mother	Weight of infant (g)				
	<1500	1500–2499	2500–3999	>4000	Total
Less than 15	0	0	0	0	0
15–19	0	3	220	1	224
20–24	4	20	579	10	613
25–29	1	16	461	16	494
30–34	3	13	443	23	482
35–39	0	9	276	19	304
40–44	1	1	123	11	136
45–49	0	0	22	0	22
50+	0	0	3	0	3
Total	9	62	2127	80	2278
%	0.4	2.7	93.4	3.5	100

Table 3.3 Live births in Shifa hospital: deliveries by birthweight. (January–April 1997: data from birth notifications)

Age of mother	Weight of infant (g)				
	<1500	1500–2499	2500–3999	>4000	Total
Less than 15	0	3	29	9	32
15–19	2	17	197	6	222
20–24	6	43	572	28	649
25–29	8	36	414	31	489
30–34	2	23	425	48	498
35–39	4	10	233	32	279
40–44	0	8	91	15	114
45–49	1	1	9	1	12
50+	0	0	0	0	0
Total	23	141	1970	161	2295
%	1.0	6.1	85.9	7.0	100

Table 3.4 Live births in Shifa hospital: deliveries by birthweight. (January–March 1997: data from hospital discharge forms)

Age of mother	Weight of infant (g)				
	<1500	1500–2499	2500–3999	>4000	Total
Less than 15	1	1	37	1	40
15–19	7	19	216	4	246
20–24	16	57	549	23	645
25–29	5	32	424	21	482
30–34	13	21	406	38	478
35–39	3	20	226	20	269
40–44	2	11	93	15	121
45–49	0	1	8	1	10
50+	0	1	3	0	4
Total	47	163	1962	123	2295
%	2.0	7.1	85.4	5.4	100

is planned with doctors and clerks at clinics and in private practices to improve the accuracy of birthweight recording.*

DISCUSSION OF CASE STUDY

What does this case study reveal specifically about Gaza and generally, about the social political and cultural context of vital statistics?

First, the Gaza population is not invisible. There are comprehensive records in two Palestinian Ministries and with the Israeli Civil Administration of all births and deaths in the population. The addresses are invisible. Is this administrative inefficiency, civil resistance or simply caution? The fact that with the exception of birthweight, other items of the birth registration are accurate would seem to indicate that this is not due entirely to administrative inefficiency.

The current intervention of revised paperwork procedures addresses the lack of coordination between agencies and ministries. While the population continues to feel it is wiser not to be easily located, improved forms will probably not affect the accuracy of the addresses given.

Several methods were used to investigate why the recording of addresses was incomplete. These ranged from discussion with members of the research team concerning hypothetical reasons and their own reasons for incomplete addresses on their ID cards, field visits to clinics and hospital registration offices and conversations with clerks. There were various explanations offered and they fall into three categories—political, economic and administrative. Some explanations were related to political circumstances. The lack of house numbers and street names during the *intifada* was a precautionary measure and although this has been partially rectified in Gaza City, there are still many areas where this continues. In addition, refugees who move outside the camps may not wish to alter their addresses on their ID cards, since there may be, in the future, compensation available for refugees of 1948.

There were also financial incentives for continuing to have an incomplete address. The two main ones mentioned were that a government employee living outside Gaza City has a transport allowance for getting to work in the city. A new address based in the city would result in the loss of this allowance. Similarly, a complete accurate address would lead to hospital bills being delivered to those who use the hospital without insurance. Hospital patients without insurance sign a commitment to pay for treatment but if they give an incomplete address the bill may never reach them.

All items on the birth registration are relatively accurate except for the addresses. This had not been a matter of concern administratively since the most important aspect of the data were the ID number and name of the individual

---

* Since the data were collected there have been other changes in Gaza—street signs have begun to go up in parts of Gaza City and an electoral register has been completed through house-to-house visits for the 1996 elections.

both for the Israeli Civil Administration and the Palestinian Ministry of the Interior. However, it was a matter of concern for the research team in order to locate their sample.

In this instance, qualitative research methods were used to discover the information pathway of birth registration data. Using field visits to clerks and health personnel, it was possible to validate information held on the register and to intervene to improve its accuracy in terms of birthweight recording.

This case study entailed understanding the situation of Palestinians living in Gaza in 1996 in terms of their physical and social vulnerabilities. The qualitative research established that, in terms of health policy, the critical missing data appropriate for intervention were the accurate recording of birthweights rather than the completion of addresses.

SOCIAL AND POLITICAL ASPECTS OF ENUMERATION

There exists a body of research carried out in different countries and hemispheres which addresses the issue of the social meaning and cultural validity of vital statistics. This general discussion reviews some of this literature in order to show how this approach is of relevance regardless of particular country or region.

It is a routine procedure to count and account for populations. This is done by carrying out censuses at regular intervals, keeping records within the health system or the education system. It is a routine part of management information systems and social security systems, both at national and regional levels. At first glance the act of counting and registering a population may seem to be a neutral activity—a prerequisite for planning, for administration, for policy development. Modern technology and in particular management information systems enable this to be achieved in an increasingly systematic manner.

However, counting is carried out within social contexts and for specific purposes. Enumeration and registration are rarely done by the community themselves, but is done to them, to us. All of us are part of databases as students, citizens, patients, tax payers, or voters. Counting is done by the agencies of the state such as Ministries of the Interior or Health or Education; by relief organisations among displaced populations and refugees (Harrell-Bond, Voutira and Leopold 1992); by researchers undertaking surveys such as the UK General Household Survey (GHS) which is carried out regularly on a national sample of households. Not only are numbers of heads counted but also aspects of people's lives, or their demographic attributes—their ethnic origin, age, address, sex, occupation, years of education are enumerated. While enumeration may bring resources to populations, the databases may simultaneously be a form of social control and sometimes the counting is recognised as a politically sensitive activity. For example, Lebanon has not carried out a national census since the 1930s as it is considered too sensitive to actually count the ethnic affiliation of the population (Deeb and Campbell 1997). As Said wrote in 1986: 'No Palestinian census exists. There is no line that can be drawn from one Palestinian to another that does not seem to interfere with the political designs of one or another state' (p. 23).

Hence, enumerating demographic attributes has a context, a purpose and lacks neutrality. Minority groups may be excluded from official statistics and health surveys either through excluding them from the population surveyed or by the statistical procedures used in analyses (Graham 1995). Using Britain as a case study, Graham has looked at the analytical procedures for the question on cohabitation in the 1991 census, and also notes the exclusion of those living in hostels, and of no fixed abode (homeless and travellers) from surveys and registers.

In the UK, direct questions on ethnic origin were only included in the GHS from 1983, and in the census from 1991. Prior to that, there had been a question on whether the head of household was born overseas, but nothing on the ethnic origin of the people in the household. This meant that the British Black population who were born in Britain were rendered invisible. Black groups lobbied for a question on ethnic origin, yet there were discussions in Parliament debating whether the question was too intrusive and the census carried out in the 1980s failed to ask about ethnicity (Booth 1988).

Counting can make marginalised people or their attributes, visible. This visibility may be 'necessary ' for the state but unwanted by groups within the population. For example, during the nineteenth and twentieth centuries within the Ottoman Empire it was common for villagers to migrate with nomadic Bedouin to avoid taxes or conscription to the Turkish army. This avoidance sometimes resulted in failure to register their land on the land register and thereby they lost their rights of ownership. Similarly, in the UK in the 1980s, many people avoided inclusion on the electoral register in order to avoid paying poll tax and thereby lost the right to vote in elections.

Enumeration and registration undeniably has many uses and are an integral part of policy, planning in the nation state. But the accuracy, desirability and meaning achieved by enumeration varies. Counting is not a neutral activity for it is embedded within particular historical and political contexts. By examining management information systems and reviewing how they are used we can gain a better understanding of the nature of MIS systems and address the problem of invisible lives.

Birth certificates may seem dry, routine sources of data. Yet as Davis (1994) in his analysis of Libyan marriage certificates 1932–1979 points out:

'The record—sometimes no more than half a small page of manuscript—is not only an artifact, a culturally specific representation of an event and not only an indicator of changed relationships and possibilities . . . the record is not simply interesting in itself, but is also a pointer to the dynamic processes of social life, of the room for manoeuvre available to Libyans and of the use which Libyans made of that room.' (pp. 204–205)

An example of this 'room for manouvre' is Hahn's (1992) fascinating analyses of the accuracy of the recording of ethnicity, 'race' and ancestry in the USA. In his examination of infant mortality from 1983 to 1985, he finds inconsistency in the coding of 'race' and ethnicity:

> '1.2% of white infants were classified differently at death than at birth. 4.3% of infants classified as black were assigned a different 'race' at death—3.6 times as many as whites . . . 30% of infants assigned a specific Hispanic origin at birth were assigned a different origin at death.' (p. 262)

Hahn also shows that the reliability of ancestral identification is problematic whether it is done by self, proxy, interviewer or funeral director (1996). He points out that 'while popular understandings of 'race' and ethnicity have not been comprehensively explored, there are indications that popular notions differ substantially from those of information-collection agencies' (1992, p. 269).

Hahn's work is a powerful appeal for a contextual cultural validity of statistics based on anthropological understandings of the meanings of ethnicity. He recommends that health surveillance systems should be periodically evaluated (1992: 271) as is done in the case study presented here. Armstrong (1986) in his historical analysis of the social construction of the biological phenomenon of infant mortality shows clearly that life and death are political, social and cultural elaborations of biological events and that registers of births and deaths are not just statistical artifacts.

Similarly, Nations and Amaral (1991) in their work in Brazil tried to bridge the gap between the simplicity of the statistics and the complexity of the social reality. They questioned the cultural validity and the contextual soundness of mortality statistics that in many countries in the South routinely exclude deaths occurring in village households, or in displaced or mobile populations. They argued that death has 'two levels of meaning the bureaucratic, official death and the personal familial loss' (p. 204).

Nations and Amaral (1991) carried out an ethnographic study of child deaths in rural Brazil and idenitified that there are incentives for village parents to report a birth—free milk, education—which make the trips into town worth it. On the other hand, there are no incentives to report a death and so these go unreported. However, without a death certificate children cannot have an official burial and are buried unofficially outside graveyards. In order to bridge the gap between the statistics and the reality, they set up two other systems in addition to the central provincial register—a survey of all households with children under 5 at the beginning and end of the year, and a team of community death reporters consisting of the midwife, the carpenter coffin maker, the storekeeper (seller of material for shrouds) and the gravedigger. At the end of the year there were nine deaths in the village of which the official registry had four, the household survey six and the popular reporters eight. Thus the alternative community-based system was more accurate than either the survey or the official registry.

Similarly, in rural South Africa in 1994, parents were very unlikely to register the deaths of their children. They were more likely to register births

(Jewkes and Wood 1998). The authors argue that vital registration was not considered vital as a means of establishing identity—other documentation would suffice and that 'Registration was seen as a *means* of achieving something else rather than an *end* in itself, which discourses of statistical and juridical importance imply' (p. 1043).

Incomplete records of birthweight or mortality make human suffering invisible. Low birthweight is a sensitive indicator of the socio-economic status of a population and is correlated with infant mortality. Underestimated mortality is a widespread problem. Maternal mortality is underestimated worldwide—sometimes no death certificates are filled in or when women die in childbirth, other reasons are given. Recent figures released by UNICEF have revised estimates of maternal mortality (Adamson 1996). In Gaza, in a move to counteract lack of accuracy in death certificates, all deaths of women of childbearing age are assumed to be possible maternal deaths until proven otherwise through investigation by the Ministry of Health. We contend that the same argument applies to life as well as death and that we need to coordinate the bureaucratic and familial levels so that statistics will be more culturally valid, accurate and humane.

Manipulation of or lack of adherence to providing information for the purpose of self-protection is not uncommon. A recent example is reported in the former Yugoslavia. During the recent war in Bosnia, health monitoring set up by the WHO was difficult to maintain both nationally and with sentinel sites partly because there was a: 'reluctance to report on the part of the local medical staff . . . some local government agencies were reluctant to part with some types of information, such as the number of ill or wounded individuals treated in a particular period, either because of a perceived possible military value or because higher authority forbade release' (Healing *et al*. 1996: 249).

Garfinkel (1967) writes about 'good' organizational reasons for 'bad' records. His work is based on the study of clinic records. He identifies 'normal natural troubles' to do with the system of reporting (in the case study, the *Kaatib* and the doctors) and the actuarial versus the therapeutic contractual uses of the records. By this, he means that the clinical records were very good concerning patient treatment but hopeless in providing technical detail which was not considered important to the patient and the staff, but useful to a researcher. He argues that treatment is the issue which concerns the clinic staff not the detail of the patient's insurer or their address.

Specifically, we may argue that there are 'good' reasons for 'bad' records in Gaza, as there were in the former Yugoslavia. Recording people's births and deaths is the main objective and this is done well. The detail of where they live is important to the individuals but not to the MIS system. Inaccurate addresses were an inconvenience to the research team who overcame it because at the local neighbourhood level there was an excellent informal system for locating people which was accessible to trusted insiders. Clinical staff knew where families lived although their addresses were not written on the health records in the clinic.

In Gaza, we are dealing with two types of power. The first is the centralised power of the state, here in the form of the Palestinian National Authority and

Israel—both of which want a record of the population, although the attributes considered important by them may be different. The second is the diffuse power of families in deciding how to deal with the birth of new family members as a private and public event, and to what extent they wish to be accountable and visible to the state (Davis 1994, citing Mason 1986).

Problems with vital registration data are particularly relevant when the nation state is in a period of transition. The case study in Gaza is drawn from the first three years of the rule of the Palestine National Authority. There is also evidence that there are problems with demographic data within the former Soviet Union as discussed by Katus, Puur and Salseus (1998) in relation to Estonia.

Katus *et al.* (1998) state that it was widely known that there were two parallel sets of statistical data—one open to the public and one only for restricted access. When the quality of data seemed poor in the past, it was assumed that the reason was due to these restrictions on data access. Katus *et al.* reveal, however, that there is 'inadequate documentation of the data sets', 'disordered statistical archives' (p. 121), and in addition a diversity of basic definitions and concepts which make comparison both within the former Soviet Union and with countries outside it highly problematic. The examples they give include definitions of live births and infant deaths where 'the definitions introduced in the Soviet Union as well as the reporting procedures did not follow the World Health Organisation's recommendations' (p. 122). This resulted in an underestimation of infant mortality. Other examples they discuss are the definitions of family and household, the comparability of marriage and divorce rates and the recording of migration. All these reflected political and social conditions and cultural meanings within the former Soviet Union which were themselves currently undergoing social transformation at this time of transition. It is critical to remember that 'statistics do not, in some mysterious way, emanate directly from the social conditions they appear to describe, but that between the two lie the asumptions, conceptions and priorities of the state and the social order, a large, complex and imperfectly functioning bureaucracy, tonnes of paper and computing machinery, and—last but not least—millions of hours of human grind'. (Government Statisticians' Collective 1993: 163).

In order to make sense of the decision making of families in Gaza one needs to consider their decisions in the context of the ongoing political and social changes, or 'events', and realise that these are not just a backdrop to their lives which provide a historic time dimension, but that they impinge on everyday decision making. The interface is complex and the interests of families and their state are not always congruent. It is here that anthropology can explore this interface and as well as explaining how social systems function, can make explicit the ways in which people use documentation to cope with suffering, oppression and hunger which are, unfortunately, part of the experience of some in all societies (Davis 1992; Hastrup 1994).

The central argument of this chapter is that vital statistics require a contextual soundness and cultural validity (Hahn 1992; Nations and Amaral 1991). They project an image of people's lives which can form the basis of regional, national and international decisions on aid budgets and health planning. But it is not enough to enumerate—the counting should be for a purpose to provide useful information so that what is made visible is human, not unwished for and not distorted.

Armstrong (1986) has pointed out that 'because the relationship between the statistics and the event is mediated by assignment the picture of 'reality' is always out of focus' (p. 230). The blurred edges are critical and need to be explored, understood and respected. Here is the place for the theory and method of social sciences to make their contribution to epidemiology. It is precisely here that qualitative research can be used to validate health surveillance data and guide policy interventions.

ACKNOWLEDGMENTS

The research reported in the case study was part of the EC funded Avicenne Initiative Grant Number 31 to evaluate and improve maternal and child health for Palestinians in Gaza. It draws heavily on the paper 'Addressing birth in Gaza using qualitative methods to improve vital registration' published in *Social Science and Medicine* 1999, 48, 833–843 by Lewando-Hundt, G., Abed, Y., Skeik, M., Beckerleg, S. and El Alem, A. which was written by the first author and editorial suggestions were received from the co-authors and referees.

REFERENCES

Abed, Y.A. (1992) Risk factors associated with prevalence of anemia among Arab children in the Gaza Strip. Unpublished PhD thesis, Johns Hopkins University.

Adamson, P. (1996) A failure of imagination. In *The Progress of Nations*. New York: UNICEF.

Armstrong, D. (1986) The invention of infant mortality. *Sociology of Health and Illness*, 8(3), 212–232.

Booth, H. (1988) Identifying ethnic origin: the past, present and future of official data production. In A. Bhat, R. Carr-Hill and S. Ohri (Eds) *Britain's Black Population*, Aldershot: Gower.

Davis, J. (1992) The anthropology of suffering. *Journal of Refugee Studies*, 5(2), 149–161.

Davis, J. (1994) Events and processes: marriages in Libya 1932–79. In K. Hastrup and P. Hervik (Eds) *Social Experience and Anthropological Knowledge* (pp. 200–223). London: Routledge.

Deeb, M. and Campbell, O. (1997) Maternal death in Lebanon. *International Journal of Obstetrics and Gynecology*.

Garfinkel, H. (1967) 'Good' organizational reasons for 'bad clinic records'. *Studies in Ethnomethodology* (pp. 186–207). Englewood Cliffs, NJ: Prentice Hall.

Gaza Health Services Research Centre (1994) *Annual Report 1994. Health Status of the Gaza Strip Population*, Ministry of Health, Palestine National Authority.

Government Statisticians' Collective (1993) How official statistics are produced: views from the inside. In M. Hammersley (Ed.) *Social Research: Philosophy, Politics and Practice* (pp. 147–165). London: Sage/Open University.

Graham, H. (1995) Diversity, inequality and official data: some problems of method and measurement in Britain, *Health and Social Care in the Community.* 3, 9–18.

Hahn, R.A. (1992) The state of federal health statistics on racial and ethnic groups. *Journal of American Medical Association*, 267(2), 268–271.

Hahn, R.A., Mulinare, J. and Teutsch S.M. (1992) Inconsistencies in coding of race and ethnicity between birth and death in US infants. A new look at Infant Mortality, 1983 Through 1985' *Journal of American Medical Association*, 267(2), 259–263.

Hahn, R.A., Truman, B.I. and Barker, N.D. (1996) Identifying ancestry: the reliability of ancestral identification in the United States by self, proxy, interviewer, and funeral director. *Epidemiology*, 7, 75–80.

Harrell-Bond, B., Voutira, E. and Leopold, M. (1992) Counting the refugees: gifts, givers, patrons and clients. *Journal of Refugee Studies*, 3(3/4), 205–225.

Hastrup K. (1994) Hunger and the hardness of facts. *Man (Ns.)*, 28, 728–739.

Healing, T.D., Drysdale, S.F., Black, M.E., Byers, Acheson, E.D., Waldman, R., Hall, S.M. and Bartlett, C.L.R. (1996) Monitoring health in the war-affected areas of the former Yugoslavia, 1992–3, *European Journal of Public Health*, 6(4), 245–251.

Jewkes R. and Wood K. (1998) Competing discourses of vital registration and personhood: perspectives from rural South Africa, *Social Science and Medicine*, 46(8),1043–1056.

Katus, K., Puur, A. and Sakeus, L. (1998) Data quality in the former Soviet Union: main hindrance is incomparability: experience of Estonia. *Migration, A European Journal of International Migration and Ethnic Relations*, 29/30/31, 119–131.

Lewando-Hundt, G. (1996) Rhetoric and reality in European cooperation with Third countries, *Journal of Social Policy and Administration*, 30(4) 368–381.

May, T. (1993) *Social Research, Issues, Methods and Process*. Buckingham: Open University Press.

The National Health Plan for the Palestinian People (1994) Jerusalem: Planning and Research Centre.

Nations, M.K. and Amaral, M.L. (1991) Flesh, blood, souls and households: cultural validity in mortality inquiry, *Medical Anthropology Quarterly*, 204–220.

Public Health Perspectives for Palestinian Refugees in a Period of Transition (1994) Proceedings of the Technical Workshop, Middle East Peace Negotiations Multilateral Working Group on Refugees, January 1994, International Course for Primary Health Care Managers at District Level in Developing Countries, Rome.

Said, E.W. (1986) *After the Last Sky, Palestinian Lives.* London: Faber and Faber.

Schnitzer, J.J. and Roy S.M. (1994) Health services under the autonomy plan. *Lancet*, 343, 1.

The Status of Health in Palestine, Annual Report (1996) Gaza: Health and Planning Directorate Statistics and Information Department.

UNDP Palestine Human Resource Development, 1996–7 (1997) Jerusalem.

UNRWA Annual Report (1996), Amman: Health Department.

Chapter 4

Cultivating Health and Preventing HIV/AIDS in the Dual Employment System of China

Shuguang Wang and Daphne Keats

Since 1978, China's urban employment system has been divided into two basic categories with different structures, the state-employment system and the *getihu* self-employment system. The self-employment (officially called *getihu*) system was adopted as the government strategy aimed at resolving the problem of massive youth unemployment in urban areas resulting from the Maoist 'Cultural Revolution'. By the end of the 1980s, most of the *getihu* were able to create jobs for themselves and rapidly entered the high-income class. At the same time, many of the *getihu* with comparatively high incomes and in independent socioeconomic situations were able to escape the official controls and conventional lifestyles imposed upon the rest of the population. The state-employment system is a traditional socioeconomic category in today's socialist China. Employees from state-owned enterprises and units enjoy more stable wages, greater benefits and better job security than the self-employed *getihu*, and their social behaviour and social relationships are more influenced by official attitudes and conventions as well as being controlled by the state-*dan wei* (unit).

This dual employment system, with its different social life situations, suggested that, generally, health among Chinese urban populations was exposed to risk at two different levels. It was therefore important to understand what role the different contexts of the two systems played in AIDS-related risk-taking sexual practices and prevention.

Cultivating Health: Cultural Perspectives on Promoting Health. Edited by M. MacLachlan.
© 2001 John Wiley & Sons Ltd.

Findings of the recent study by Wang (1998) which will be presented in this chapter show a profile of social lifestyles among the *getihu* which are at risk for exposure to AIDS and other sexually transmitted diseases, revealing a new frontier for programmes in Chinese public health. The experiences of a group of AIDS and STD sufferers are shown in the following case studies.

CASE STUDIES*

Fei Jiang is a member of the new social class of self-employed in China, the *getihu*. He is HIV positive. Fei Jiang grew up in a working-class family in the city of Chengdu in the Sichuan Province of South Western China. His father was a private tricycle operator, earning a meagre living pedalling for fares around the city. His mother was a housewife. Neither his father nor his mother had attended school. The family circumstances were poor and under-privileged. The family lived outside the state-*dan wei* (state-unit) living area and were known as 'urban street residents'. Fei himself became a 'street boy' or 'street corner boy' in 1989. As a street boy living in a family of low economic status Fei was never expected to obtain a higher level of education or a good job. He started selling cigarettes along the streets while he was still at school.

From this humble background Fei grew up to become a *getihu* engaged in a successful trans-regional business. He became a long-distance bus driver and engaged in the sale of clothing and electrical equipment across the region. As the business developed, Fei travelled widely, often going as far as Hong Kong, Thailand and Burma. By the age of twenty-seven, and unmarried, he had become a 'rich boss'.

Fei described the active social life he led as a rich *getihu*:

> 'Almost every day my friends and I go out to various public places for entertain-ment. I am now a rich boss, so I can spend more time in karaoke bars and discos together with my friends. We like eating, drinking, talking, dancing and playing games at different places, and trying the different lifestyles, we spend every day like this.

Friends were all-important sources for entertainment, but also for providing sexual experiences. Fei says:

> 'Friends always introduce different places and girls to me. We often get together to play Mar Jiang (Mah Jong), watch pornographic video tapes and go to karaoke bars. We sometimes exchange our casual sexual partners, and practise different sexual intercourse, such as oral sex, anal sex, toy sex, etc.'

Fei was first diagnosed with genital herpes three years previously, but this did not prevent him continuing with his sexual activities. When the treatment alleviated his symptoms, he ceased it and within a short time he was diagnosed

---

* Real names have not been used.

as HIV positive. The combination of a lack of supportive treatment, his own ignorance and sense of shame led him to try to treat himself. He says:

'I got the genital herpes infection in 1993. I stopped my treatment when the symptoms were alleviated. I have been to Hong Kong, Thailand and Burma both for business and just for travelling. It was during this period that I was diagnosed as HIV positive. I do not have a history of drug use, so it was probably transmitted by my sexual life with prostitutes. I think that this is retribution for my sexual life, because no matter where I had been I went to snooker, discos, and massage rooms very often. I spend almost all of my money playing "cats" [having sex with prostitutes]. Before, I did not know what HIV/AIDS was at all, even now I still have little knowledge of it. Also, I can get very little advice or treatment suggestions from doctors in the Center for AIDS Control and Prevention of Chengdu, state hospitals, and private STD clinics. I have to treat it by myself. I have bought many medicines, such as "Jieeryin", "3-Star 168-Jieyinlin", and "miemiaolin" etc. I also went to see the Chinese medical doctors at the University of Chinese Medical Sciences.'

Fei Jiang's case was one of a group of ten in-depth case studies of STD and AIDS sufferers interviewed as part of Wang's study of knowledge, attitudes and behaviour to STD and AIDS among 400 young men in Sichuan Province. The study included 200 who were self-employed (*getihu*) and 200 employed in the state-*dan wei* system. The ten case studies included seven STD patients, of whom five were *getihu* and two non-*getihu*, and three HIV-positive patients who were all *getihu*.

Fei Jiang's experiences are similar to those of many *getihu* who worked their way from poor circumstances into a *getihu*'s sub-cultural context and a high risk lifestyle. Both the STD and AIDS sufferers interviewed revealed a similar lack of knowledge as to the nature of the AIDS infection. That AIDS was a disease of foreigners only, and that it was confined to homosexuals was their common belief. One STD sufferer said,

'I am not so clear about what AIDS is, I have only heard this word from my friends. I know it is a disease of homosexuals overseas, probably this disease has got something to do with abnormal sex among homosexuals. I had no idea how people could catch AIDS. I was told that this disease can be transmitted among homosexuals.' (Liu, *getihu*)

Another,

'HIV/AIDS is a most serious cancer, but I did not worry about it, as I did not think that I had any chance to catch it because I had no contact with homosexuals or foreigners.' (Song Xiang, *getihu*)

AIDS was associated with the lifestyles of Western countries:

'Do you know how people call AIDS? It is called "high-grade STD", that means AIDS is related to people who are in Western countries, and who are rich with extra money to take drugs and enjoy sexual freedom. So AIDS is the result of Western civilisation, rather than a disease which could be epidemic in developing countries.' (Zhen Yong, *getihu*)

A non-*getihu* STD sufferer reflected the official emphasis on morality:

'I remember once that the newspaper mentioned that AIDS is the disease which is associated with people who have sex with foreigners, particularly having sex with homosexuals, so AIDS is certainly seen as a disease related to immoral sexual behaviour, in particular abnormal sexual behaviour.' (Cheng Zhixiao, non-*getihu*)

Two HIV positive sufferers revealed the same lack of knowledge but continued to have casual sex with prostitutes because they were unaware that they, in turn, were at risk. Like Fei Jiang, they also travelled widely, to the coastal cities and about the country.

'I had heard about AIDS before, but I did not know what the disease was. I remember one of my friends told me that AIDS is related to homosexuality and to the taking of drugs. I often have sex with prostitutes in coastal cities, however I did not know that I could catch HIV by having casual sex with prostitutes. I thought that I am not homosexual, so I should not be at risk from HIV/AIDS infection.' (Laio Jingling, *getihu*)

'I started to know some information about STD from my friends when they were infected. They said that the street girls in the towns were more dangerous because they had too many sex partners each day. So often I had relation with the girls in the country. I know little about HIV before catching HIV. I guessed it was the disease for foreigners, and since our Chinese are not interested in homosexuals, I thought we will not be infected.' (Xie Gang, *getihu*)

Involvement in their social contexts was important for the getihu for both pleasure and business contacts, but also as a source of sexual partners:

'Karaoke bars and discos are the most gravitational places for me. If it is possible, I'd like to spend more free time in these places. There, I can meet my friends, and enjoy eating, drinking, and dancing, and also looking for new girl friends.' (Du Ke, *getihu*)

'In the past, as a street boy, I used to wonder where I could go to meet friends and spend time. Now I can set up our offices in the hotels, and spend our spare time in restaurants, café rooms, ballrooms, hotel lobbies and snookers halls, etc. These places are becoming the *getihu*'s new places both for carrying on their businesses and entertainment. They also go there to look for sexual partners and other consumption activities in these public places.' (Song Xiang, *getihu*).

'I can say that my whole life has been changed since I engaged in the *getihu* economy, my life is much different from the past. Before I had to spend all of my free time at home, because my low income was not enough to do any outside recreational consumption. Now the income from my business not only supports my family but also my widespread social activities and recreational life . I often meet my business friends and together we play cards, snooker (gambling), go to restaurants, karaoke bars, and saunas. I think that in my parents' and my own past life we all suffered too much and I don't want to recall it. Now, my life has been changed, so I have no reason why not to enjoy my life as much as I can.' (Liu Jayiu., *getihu*)

Two non-*getihu* STD sufferers reflected their change of lifestyles because of their involvement in *getihu* socioeconomic contexts:

'Since I decided to "go down to the sea" [i.e. engage in non-governmental business], meeting with the *getihu* is my everyday life. I must enter into their society both in business relations and lifestyles if I want to be successful in my own business. In other words, I must go to the *getihu*'s companies, shops, street corners, and various recreational places to further develop new relations of socio-business. For many State-employed people, you know, they do not like to get involved in the *getihu*'s business and their lifestyles, due to conventional values and beliefs. But, as a business man, you know, Chinese business is based more on trust and friendship than on business rules, therefore, I must establish the business interpersonal networks with them. Also, I must do what they do and go where they go, such as the places of karaoke bars, coffee rooms, massage parlours and so on.' (Cheng Zhixao, non-*getihu*)

'Although I am still counted as a member of the state-owned enterprise, I "go down to the sea" and am involved in private businesses. This also signals that I am an individual businessman even though I do not hold a formal license. In fact, I am not very much different from the *getihu*. My household register number is still kept in the state-*dan wei*, but my wages have already been stopped. Now I live on the income from my business. Most of my friends are *getihu*, we often go together for drinking, dancing, playing cards, gambling, and meeting girls. I think the purpose of my life is to get more money and better business opportunities. So it is hard to imagine what I would have done if I hadn't decided to do private business and entered into the *getihu*'s networks and their entertainment spaces.' (Zhang Feng, non-*getihu*)

THEORETICAL PERSPECTIVE: SEXUAL PRACTICE AND SOCIAL-CULTURAL CONTEXTS

The personal experiences in the narratives from Fei Jiang and the other cases show that the society of their existence is not constituted as a homogeneous whole. The social position, employment sectors and occupation status differ significantly between the self-employed *getihu* and the non-*getihu* employed by the state-*dan wei*. The differences in their social position and social life were generated by the dual social/class structure and employment system of Chinese urban society. This dual social structure determines how individual social life is collectively composed of class structure and power relations, while individuals' personal social existence and health-related lifestyles operate through their own social group and contexts. As the narratives from the above cases illustrate, the self-employed's social background led to their collective involvement in subcultural social activities and group networks, and their knowledge about HIV-related risk-taking issues and socio-sexual practices was significantly associated with their involvement in their socio-subcultural contexts. This implies a social structure (class) and collective agency of individual sexual behaviour.

Sexuality associated with personal social life history, cultural patterns and social relationships has been documented in early academic research in Western countries, such as Freud (1905/1930), Marcuse (1955) and Malinowski (1927, 1932, 1960). In 'frame theories of sexuality' (Gagnon and Simon 1974), human sexuality was emphasised as socially scripted, and socially constructed. Sexuality was also regarded as a social structure within the theoretical tradition of Durkheim, structuralist Marxism and post-structuralism which was widely used as a theoretical frame to analyse the social system, politics, history and cultural symbolic system in relation to sexual practice (Ma 1990; Wuthnow, Bergesen and Kurzweil 1984).

From the point of view of social structuralism, the social frames of sexuality, both as practice and social relations, are taken from relevant social or historical structural domains (Rubin 1975), while sexual practices can be constructed as class sexuality, employment sexuality (Pringle 1988), and organisation sexuality (Hearn and Parkin 1987).

The post-structuralist, Foucault, discussed the particular dimension of knowledge and power related to sexuality. In his first volume of *The History of Sexuality* (1978) Foucault stresses that the relation of sex to power is rooted in its social system. According to Foucault, 'discourses' play an important role in the constitution of mechanisms for the social control of bodies and sex. The relations between sexuality and power are predicted in details within the social system, such as public discourses, institutions, our bodies, etc. Sexuality is not only to show the power network, but also 'it appears rather as an especially dense transfer point for relations of power' (1978: 103). In this regard, for Foucault, 'sexuality is not the most intractable element in power relations, but rather as one of those endowed with the greatest instrumentality'. The relevant morality and norms, professional knowledge and institutions will be used to control covert sexual behaviour, when sexuality becomes a topic of public discourse, especially when sexual behaviour as an 'issue' is incorporated into the public discourse. In general, Foucault's work on sexuality stressed the theoretical nature of the social construction of sexuality, and his social constructionist framework is being increasingly utilised by historians and sociologists (Wuthnow *et al.* 1984).

However, in cross-cultural research with AIDS-related sexual behaviour, broad differences in values, beliefs and practices within different sexual cultures have been documented in the United States (see, for example, Gagnon 1989; Abramson 1988; Abramson and Herdt 1990; Carballo *et al.* 1989; Herdt and Stoller 1990), in Africa (see, for example, MacLachlan 1997; DiClemente, Forrest and Mickler 1990; DiClemente, Zorn and Temoshok 1987; Orubuloye *et al.* 1994; Scott and Mercer 1994), the United Kingdom (see, for example, Fitzpatrick, Boulton and Hart 1989; Watney 1990), and Australia (see, for example, Kippax *et al.* 1990, 1992, 1993; McCamish and Najman 1995). The different and complex settings of sexual culture are an important stand point for understanding and regulating sexual behaviour in different sociocultural contexts. Although sexual culture is shown by an individual's social role, attitude and behaviour, it is also the expression of the collectivity (Herdt and Abramson 1990; Herdt, Parker and Carballo 1991; Parker, Herdt and Carballo 1991; Kippax *et al.* 1993). Further, cross-cultural research with AIDS-related issues has emphasised the differences in sexual practices within different cultures, societies, and groups, and, especially in the case of AIDS, strongly suggests the interplay between risk-taking behaviour among members of a group and the group's social class and cultural context

(MacLachlan 1997; Parker *et al.* 1991; Carael, Cleland and Deheneffe 1992; Helman 1990).

In addition, in the social contextual perspective of sexuality, sexuality is not constituted simply within social structure, agency and social process but is deeply embedded in social and historical practice itself (Kippax *et al.* 1993). Empirical evidence from the studies of Kippa *et al.* (1990, 1992, 1993) in Australia indicate that sexual practice is a collective agency which is historically enacted. Other research in the USA, such as by Blaxter (1990), Williams (1995) and Illsley (1980) on the relationship between social/class contexts and health practices also suggests that the interrelation of class and health behaviour is crucial to identify the collective behaviour of the group with health-related risk-taking practices at different sociocultural levels.

Recent Chinese research has also shown relationships between different sexual practice and social structures. As the studies by Song (1991), Ruan (1991), Xiao (1993), Shiao (1987, 1992), and Wang (1989) indicate, Chinese conventional sexual beliefs, values and practices are not only impacted by sociocultural development and system restructuring, but are also constructed within different social structures. In Mao's time, although some accepted conventional and traditional practices such as polygamy, concubinage and prostitution were identified as illegal and removed, the government neverthe-less adopted as its own the quasi-traditional norms of sexual behaviour, and incorporated them into both law and social relations in ways that conformed to Party ideology. Thus pre-marital virginity, married fidelity (actually a wife's fidelity to her husband) and widowed fidelity were encouraged exten-sively. Having more than one pre-marital partner (without sexual contact), pre-marital sexual behaviour, extra-marital sexual relations, unmarried unions and divorce were labelled as 'shameless', 'degrading', 'immoral', and 'illicit'. Therefore, such behaviour was seen as a serious issue and an obstacle to a person employed in a state-*dan wei* in terms of promoting his occupational position, affecting his income growth and political progress.

In the post-Mao era, along with the development of the Chinese *Shixiang jiefang yundong* (ideological liberation movement) and social system reform, people's ideologies, including sexual values, have been released to some extent from the bind of Chinese sociocultural morality. This was particularly so for the young *getihu* who live outside the state-*dan wei* system and who have a more open attitude toward sex. At the same time, however, they are also facing a series of 'issues' regarding their sexual practices. For example, having sex with prostitutes has become more prevalent, multiple sexual partnerships and divorce have dramatically increased and practices which put them at risk of HIV/AIDS and other STDs have become widespread. In response to this, the government has attempted to deal with the 'sexual issues' through public 'sexual moral and knowledge education'. However, to a very large extent, government strategy can only be effectively carried out among the non-*getihu* population within the state-*dan wei* system. In this regard, many of the non-*getihu* population are still more likely to adopt conventional norms with sexual practices unless they are away from the state-*dan wei* controlling system

World-wide studies of STD/AIDS epidemiology have shown that young people were more likely to take greater risks for STD and HIV/AIDS infection due to socio-psycho-sexual factors (Manoff 1989; Gao 1991; Stevenson *et al*. 1992; Moore, Rosenthal and Mitchell 1996). Also, consistent with this tendency, a nation-wide survey of China's STD epidemic from 1991 to 1996 (Xu and Shao 1996) showed that 92.8% of STD cases were young people aged 20 to 39. However, the rapid increase of STD and HIV/AIDS cases in the Chinese youth population was significantly associated with special social and economic categories such as the young self-employed *getihu* (Xu and Shao 1996; Zheng 1997).

Analysis of the *getihu*'s unconventional socio-sexual practices (see, for example, Gil *et al*. 1994, 1996; Xiao 1993; Shiao 1987, 1992; Guo 1985; Pien 1989; Wang 1998; Gao and Zhang 1991; Yu 1989; Zhao and Lu, 1985) indicated that the differences between the *getihu* and the non-*etihu* were generated by the dual social/class structure of Chinese urban society. Massive system reform, changes in the social control system, the rapid development of the urban marketing economy, and wide-ranging individual business travel allowed self-employed young people to have more opportunities to escape the tight conventional social and economic control imposed on the rest of the population, and further, most of them were able to adopt unconventional sexual practices.

Wu and Wu (1982, 1983), Cheng (1991) and Wang (1986a,b, 1987) stressed collective agency for the development of a subcultural group of unconventional sexual values, beliefs and practices among self-employed young people from a social psychological approach. Also social contextual views of sexual practice in the research by Wang (1998) and Wang, Gao and Zhao (1998) indicate that the collective vulnerability for HIV among the self-employed *getihu* was not only associated with their exposure to risk-taking sexual practice but also constructed by their specific socio-cultural context, the interrelation of class (structure), sexual life history and social-historical constitution of sexuality within China's dual social system. The different socio-sexual practices among Chinese populations were moderated by their involvement in different socio-cultural contexts, and suggested that the impact of China's employment system was an important social dimension for AIDS-related sexual practices and their prevention among Chinese.

INSIGHTS FROM RESEARCH: CHINA'S DUAL SOCIAL SYSTEM AND *GETIHU* SOCIAL CONTEXTUAL MEANINGS FOR STD/AIDS RISK

By mid-1997 over 300 000 cases of HIV/AIDS had occurred in China, and it has been estimated that by the year 2000 the total will have reached over a million if the present trend continues (Zheng 1997). During the period 1990–1997 the highest incidence of HIV/AIDS cases (661 average per year) was found among the self-employed *getihu* population (Xu and Shao 1998).

As shown in Table 4.1, data from the study by Wang (1998) indicates that the *getihu* were more likely than the non-*getihu* to spend much of their money in their own social group, for example in 'low social level contexts' ($F_{(1,398)} = 48.74$, $p < 0.001$) (such as street karaoke bars, tea rooms, coffee rooms, massage rooms, saunas, discos, the *getihu* clubs, the *getihu* corners, and so on); 'informal *getihu*'s group activities ($F_{(1,241)} = 44.61$, $p < 0.001$), and the *getihu*'s business activities ($F_{(1,304)} = 155.20$, $p < 0.001$) (see Table 4.1). The *getihu*'s involvement in their own socio-geographic networks suggested that this allowed them to adopt collective and unconventional beliefs in regard to socio-sexual practices.

Table 4.1 Differences between the *getihu* group and state employed group with regard to their level of involvement in different social/cultural contexts[a]

Analysis of variance (F-values)	LSLC		HSLC		IGSA		FGSA		IPB	
	Self-emp.	State-emp.	Self-emp.	State-emp.	Self-emp.	State-emp.	Self-emp.	State-emp.	Self-emp.	State-emp.
N	200	200	162	81	196	148	101	197	199	107
Mean	16.4	8.9	4.53	0.65	5.82	1.74	0.3	5.0	6.15	0.71
SD	8.47	3.55	6.23	1.25	2.90	1.65	0.6	1.8	3.10	1.61
F-value	$F_{(1,398)} = 48.74$		$F_{(1,241)} = 44.61$		$F_{(1,342)} = 85.40$		$F_{(1,296)} = 129.80$		$F_{(1,304)} = 155.20$	
p (Significance level)	<0.001		<0.001		<0.001		<0.001		<0.001	

Source: Wang (1998).
Self-emp. is self-employed group: State-emp. is state-ownership employed group.

LSLC is low social level context (refers to places with a low level in terms of management, conditions and services, such as street karaoke bars, tea rooms, coffee rooms, massage rooms, discos, and so on).

HSLC is high social level context (refers to places with a high level in terms of the management, conditions and service, such as luxury tea houses, high-grade karaoke bars, saunas and massage rooms in star hotels and other public places).

IGSA is informal group social activities.

FGSA is formal group social activities.

IPB is individual private business.

[a] Level of involvement was scored 1 if response was 'seldom' for subject's involvement in LSLC, HSLC, IGSA, FGSA and IBP; 2 if response was 'sometimes'; 3 if response was 'often'; 4 if response was 'always'. The level of involvement score ranged from 4 to 34 with a mean of 13.38 and a standard deviation of 4.20 for subjects' involvement in their social and cultural contexts.

It was also found from this research (Wang 1998) that the *getihu* were more likely than the non-*getihu* to receive unreliable and inaccurate information on AIDS and engage in unprotected sex with casual partners. In addition, data in Wang (1998)'s study further indicated that because of their broad involvement in urban socio-geographic recreational activities and places, the *getihu* tended to have sexual contacts with more than one sexual partner in various parts of the country, particularly in coastal cities and border areas. Although there was also a fairly low level of condom use among people in the non-*getihu* group, they were less exposed to risk because their sexual activities continued to be strongly influenced by conventional morality and official restrictions.

Data from Gil, Wang and Anderson (1994, 1996) shows that in China most information on AIDS from mainstream sources has moralistic or punitive associations while failing to provide adequate guidance on safe sex. In the non-*getihu* the tendency was to construct their beliefs about HIV as 'morality-bound diseases', they therefore were more likely than the *getihu* people to think that AIDS was related to stigma, perverse sexual practices, and immoral sexual behaviour. However, the collective representation with HIV/AIDS among the *getihu* was significantly different. Among the *getihu* people HIV/AIDS was more likely to be explained and interpreted as a 'disease of homosexuals or foreigners', a 'high-grade STD' or 'a disease of the rich in Western countries', rather than as a morally bound disease. This difference in metaphor suggests that those self-employed *getihu* exposed to the impact of HIV-related risk-taking sexual practices and the punitive strategies of conventional morality for unconventional sexual behaviour have had to seek support from informal sources such as interpersonal communications within their socio-sexual networks, commercial advertisements in the informal press and informal printed booklets (illegally printed pornographic magazines), rather than from more accurate formal information sources. Moreover, findings from Wang's (1998) study showed that there was a significant relationship between the involvement of the *getihu* in various subcultural socioeconomic groups and their information patterns and accuracy of knowledge about sexually transmitted diseases and AIDS. The *getihu* who had comparatively frequent contact with members of low socioeconomic groups and their activities were more likely to receive unreliable or inadequate information on AIDS than those who moved in higher social level contexts.

The data analysis in Table 4.2 presents a picture of a difference between the *getihu* and the non-*getihu* in their approach to safe and unsafe sexual practices. The major findings of this analysis indicate that most members of the *getihu* group were more likely than the non-*getihu* group to engage in risk-taking sexual behaviour. The statistical significance indicates that risk-taking sexual behaviour among the *getihu* group was related to their multiple sexual activities with more than one casual sexual partner within an extensive socio-geographic area, without using condoms or with a very low rate of condom use.

Further data analysis showed how knowledge, beliefs and safe/unsafe sexual behaviour were moderated by the contextual involvement of the *getihu*. Multiple regression analysis of the full model in Table 4.3 indicates that involvement in the lower social level contexts among those self-employed people was the strongest predictor in all variables (socio-demographic, geographic, contextual, knowledge and psychological risk-taking factors) in regard to their adopting unsafe sexual behaviour.

The findings suggest that these *getihu* were more likely than other respondents to reveal a connection between their unreliable knowledge about AIDS, psychological risk-taking tendency and risk-taking sexual practices due to their involvement in the lower level social contexts. In other words, as the narratives of Fei Jiang and other cases have shown, unreliable knowledge of AIDS and adoption of unsafe sexual behaviour were significantly associated with frequent involvement in the collective activities within various *getihus'* socio-geographic spaces and subculture such as street

Table 4.2 Sexual partners and sexual practices

Sexual partners and sexual practices (n = 266)	Frequency		Chi-square test (single variable test)		
	Getihu	Non-*getihu*	χ^2	df	p
(1) Having sex with more than one sexual partner	164	102	6.66	1	<0.01
(2) Types of sexual relationship among subjects who have more than one regular sexual partner					
Regular sexual partners (no payment)	11	19	9.16	1	<0.01
Regular sexual partners (no payment)	23	8	47.87	1	<0.01
Casual sexual partners (no payment)	49	36	6.61	1	<0.02
Casual sexual partners (payment)	13	8	5.05	1	<0.05
Regular (payment) + casual (payment)	68	31	18.66	1	<0.01
(3) Regions for contact with more than one sexual partners					
Inner city	57	45	5.73	1	<0.02
Suburbs	26	21	2.15	1	n.s.
Other provinces or coastal cities	16	13	1.25	1	n.s.
Border areas[a]	14	2	–		–
Hong Kong or overseas[a]	9	0	–		–
Other combined options	42	20	11.52	1	<0.01
(4) Sexual repertoire (genital–vaginal sex[b] + follows)[c]					
O/G + MM	19	25	3.34	1	n.s.
O/G + MM + O/V + SEL	16	18	0.02	1	n.s.
O/G + O/V + O/A + G/A + MM + MIT + SEB	51	23	28.55	1	<0.01
O/A + O/V + MM + MIT + SEB	41	21	21.70	1	<0.01
O/A + O/V + MIT	23	9	30.31	1	<0.01
O/A + MM + SEB	14	6	27.10	1	<0.01
(5) Never/quite rarely use a condom when having sex	141	55	25.75	1	<0.01
	(89.0%)	(53.9%)			

Source: Wang (1998).
[a] Excluded from the analysis because expected frequency is less than 5.
[b] Data in the study show that all subjects who report they have sexual behaviour engaged in genital-sexual practice.
[c] O/G is oral–genital sex; O/V is oral–vaginal sex; O/A is oral–anal sex; MM is mutual masturbation; MIT is massage instrument and toy sex; SEB is special experience sex involving sex-related bleeding (modes of skin damage); and SEL is special experience sex involving a little related bleeding.

discos, karaoke bars, massage rooms, tea houses, pool and snooker halls, video arcades and *getihu* street corners. In these socio-geographic spaces and the *getihu*'s sub-cultural groups, AIDS was conventionalised by their existing schemata of the *getihu* subcultural beliefs and values as an unfamiliar and low-risk social phenomenon.

Individual knowledge, beliefs and information about AIDS (e.g. it is a 'disease of homosexuals or foreigners', 'high-grade STD' or 'a disease of the

Table 4.3 Multiple regression models: the correlation between independent variables (contextual, demographic/geographic, knowledge, and psychological risk-taking) and safe/unsafe sexual behaviour within self-employed people and state-employed people ($n = 359$)[a]

	Dependent variables							
	Unsafe sex				Safe sex			
Independent variables	Self-employment ($n = 186$)		State-employment ($n = 173$)		Self-employment ($n = 186$)		State-employment ($n = 173$)	
	β	p	β	p	β	p	β	p
Locale	−0.1077	***	−0.2407	***	−0.2807	***	0.1634	***
Age	0.0523		0.0238		0.0343	*	−0.0116	
Occupation	−0.1928	***	−0.0397		0.1728	***	0.0254	
Education	−0.1224	**	−0.0129		0.0424	*	−0.0301	
Income	−0.2118	***	0.2118	*	0.2118	***	0.0322	
Low social level contacts	0.2743	***	0.1223	***	−0.0643	**	−0.1872	***
High social level contexts	−0.1002		0.0412		0.3942	***	0.0371	
Informal group activities	0.2309	**	0.0486	***	0.1186	**	−0.1773	**
Formal group activities	0.0321	**	−0.0913	*	0.0216		0.1571	***
Individual private business	0.1354	*	0.0813	*	0.614	**	−0.1343	**
Knowledge about safe-sex	−0.1363	**	−0.0321		0.1647	***	0.0402	
Knowledge about risk-sex	−0.0344		0.0667	*	0.0737	***	0.0271	
Psychological risk-taking	0.1480	*	0.1834	***	−0.2054	**	−0.0863	**
	Adj. $R^2 = 24.2\%$ $F_{(13,344)} = 10.90$ $p < 0.001$		Adj. $R^2 = 16.6\%$ $F_{(13,344)} = 13.77$ $p < 0.001$		Adj. $R^2 = 20.9\%$ $F_{(13,344)} = 16.21$ $p < 0.001$		Adj. $R^2 = 16.39\%$ $F_{(13,344)} = 14.20$ $p < 0.001$	

Source: Wang (1998).

Notes:
[a] Case numbers are those who report they have sexual behaviour among total 400 subjects.
β Standardised regression coefficient (Beta).
* < 0.01 ** < 0.001 *** < 0.0001.
Adj. R^2: Adjusted R^2.

rich in Western countries' which imply the non-relevance to their own self) among these *getihu* groups were collectively formed and collectively maintained explanations which supported and encouraged their unconventional sexual practices. Consequently, the *getihus'* sub-cultural contexts affected not only their risk-taking sexual practice for HIV infection but also the way the public responds to sexual health education messages.

As shown in the narratives of the non-*getihu* cases, with the restructuring of China's social system and the development of the market economy, the *getihu's* self-employed socioeconomic patterns and subculture group are extending rapidly. In addition, as a massive young rural population is now entering the urban *getihu* labour market, and more of the state-ownership employed populations are laid off and have to 'go down to the sea' (become involved in the *getihus'* business), the *getihu* self-employed socio-cultural context is becoming the mainstream of socio-economic life among today's Chinese population. By implication, it is likely that more and more individuals will be involved not only in the self-employed people's socio-economic and subcultural contexts but also in their unconventional socio-psycho-sexual practices with attendant risks of STD and HIV/AIDS.

However, evidence from this study and other relevant research (see, for example, Gil, Wang and Anderson 1996: Wang 1998; Wang, Gao and Zhao 1998) has shown that mainstream prevention messages are rarely deployed in the socio-geographic contexts to which the *getihu* and their sexual partners gravitate. This creates dilemmas for intervention in the HIV epidemic and strongly suggests that HIV prevention strategies need to cross the socioeconomic and sociocultural divide created by the dual employment structure.

RECOMMENDATIONS: A NEW FRONTIER FOR CHINA'S PUBLIC HEALTH AND STD/AIDS PREVENTION

Although the Chinese government has launched many anti-HIV/AIDS epidemic campaigns, the rapid increase in the proportion of the *getihu* population among HIV/AIDS sufferers has shown the difficulty in both understanding the risk-taking sexual practices among the *getihu* and adopting appropriate prevention strategies. In particular, in the current government public health education and promotion, research is sadly lacking in understanding the fundamental characteristics of the dual system in contemporary China. As the experiences of Fei Jiang and the other cases illustrate, they were not able to break the connection between their social role of being in the *getihu* self-employed class and their subcultural contexts. This suggests that HIV prevention messages should be designed to reach into the *getihu*'s socio-subcultural geographic contexts. To achieve this the following strategies should be considered:

(1) Because the sexual practices among self-employed *getihu* differ from state-employed non-*getihu*, special intervention strategies with sexual health education and HIV/AIDS prevention programs which can reach self-employed populations should be developed within the various social networks and social contexts to which the *getihu* and their sexual partners gravitate. That means reaching into those consumer and recreation places where Fei Jiang and his friends frequently congregate such as karaoke bars, coffee rooms, massage rooms, tea houses, public bathing pools, and barbershops, which act as fronts for their socio-sexual activities.

(2) Multi-faceted intervention strategies including both official information sectors and informal social support from the *getihus'* own sectors should be used to promote sexual health education and risk reduction. Clear effects were noted in Wang (1998)'s study that legitimate and official information sources of sexual education information could be obtained through informal social support sectors such as booklets containing information on business, entertainment and health which were informally printed and delivered among those *getihu* who were

involved in higher social level contexts. This informal printed matter plays an important role as a major sector of informal social support in HIV-related information interpretation, circulation and communication in the *getihu* population. It is therefore suggested that informal printed matter with HIV-related information can be used within the informal social support sectors to improve mainstream information. When this printed matter is improved and modified as formal booklets and pamphlets with legitimate knowledge, they can be distributed more widely into the *getihus'* socio-subcultural geographic contexts.

(3)   Legitimate knowledge of safe/unsafe sex should be deployed in private STD clinics, and in the posters advertising these clinics. In contemporary China, shame and social stigma concerning STD and AIDS are still common. STD and HIV/AIDS are emphasised as morality-bound diseases in conventional values and official ideology, and in the campaigns against prostitutes and their clients, legal action replaced health education and social support with adequate information. Therefore, most individuals, in both urban and rural areas, when infected by STD and HIV, prefer to seek treatment in private STD clinics in order to avoid any official record of having a sexually transmitted disease (Kuang and Teng 1989; Dalian STD Anti-Epidemic Institute 1989). However, the narratives from these cases' experience of being STD/HIV sufferers and seeking treatment show that there was a great lack of adequate or even general information about STD and HIV. Quantitative data analysis also confirmed that most STD and HIV sufferers can obtain very little reliable knowledge and adequate advice from non-official STD clinic sectors (Wang 1998). China's public health workers should realise that non-official health sectors have played a more important role with AIDS-related prevention in self-employed *getihu* populations. In today's China, AIDS prevention needs to develop more education programs to increase information within the non-official health service sectors, especially the private STD clinics, due to the mainstream information sectors facing the impact of changes in the social system.

(4)   More work on STD/AIDS prevention should be developed within the national family planning organisation. The Family Planning Organisation is one of the largest government organisations on health and family planning, and can provide the connection with the *getihu* social groups. The family planning campaign about condom use should also play a role in STD/AIDS prevention, not only for population control. The intervention strategies of AIDS need to be integrated extensively within policies made by the family planning institutes, and AIDS-related preventive work should be supported and carried out within the networks for family planning.

(5)   As the major source of information on STD/AIDS-related risks, the official mass media should disseminate more factual knowledge about safe and unsafe sex, not only information on the traditional sexual morality and psychologically threatening messages related to unconventional sexual practices with the attendant risk of STD/AIDS. The strategy of stressing a simple moralistic, frightening and punitive

perspective was confirmed as unsuccessful in regard to changing risk-taking sexual behaviour among young Chinese people. As a whole, the findings from current research suggest that the Chinese government should work to establish an understanding that sexual practice is not a uniform or isomorphous practice in the population, and move away from a simple and moralistic or punitive perspective, and finally develop an appropriate intervention strategy to reduce those risk factors within the dual social system of China.

REFERENCES

Abramson, P.R. (1988) Sexual assessment and the epidemiology of AIDS. *The Journal of Sex Research*, 25, 323–346.

Abramson, P.R. and Herdt, G. (1990) The assessment of sexual practices relevant to the transmission of AIDS: A global perspective. *The Journal of Sex Research*, 27, 215–232.

Blaxter, M. (1990) *Health and Lifestyles*. London: Routledge.

Carael, M., Cleland, J. and Deheneffe, J. C. (1992) Research on sexual behaviour that transmits HIV: The GPA/WHO collaborative surveys—preliminary findings. In T. Dgson (Ed.) *Sexual Behaviour and Networking*. USA: International University for the Scientific Study of Population.

Carballo, M., Cleland, J., Carael, M. and Albrecht, G. (1989) A cross national study of patterns of sexual behaviour. *The Journal of Sex Research*, 26(3), 287–290.

Cheng, J.K. (1991) Psychological risk-taking factors and health-related behaviour. *The Collected Papers for Population and Health (China-Hube)*, 14(2), 7–9.

Dalian STD Anti-epidemic Institute (DSAI) (1989) STDs under-reports are extremely universal phenomenon. In Department of Anti-Epidemic and prevention of Minister of Public Health of China (Eds) *The Collected Papers for STD Preventive Work and Research Report*.

DiClemente, R.J., Forrest, K.A. and Mickler, S. (1990) College students' knowledge and attitudes about AIDS and changes in HIV preventive behaviours. *AIDS Education and Prevention*, 2, 201–212.

DiClemente, R.J., Zorn, J. and Temoshok, L. (1987) The association of gender, ethnicity and length of residence in the bay area to adolescents' knowledge and attitudes about AIDS. *Journal of Applied Social Psychology*, 17, 30–216.

Fitzpatrick, R., Boulton, M. and Hart, G. (1989) Gay men's sexual behaviour in response to AIDS: Insights and problems, In P. Aggleton, P. Davies and G. Hart (Eds) *AIDS: Social representations, social practices*. Lewes: Falmer Press.

Foucault, M. (1990 [1978]) *The History of Sexuality, Vol. 1: An introduction*. (R. Hurley, Trans.). New York: Vintage Books (original work published 1978).

Freud, S. (1953) [1905] Three essays on the theory of sexuality. In *Complete Psychological Works*, Standard edn, Vol. 7. London: Hogarth.

Freud, S. (1963) [1930] *Civilization and Discontents* (J. Riviere, Rev. and J. Strachey, Trans.). London: Hogarth (original work published 1930).

Gagnon, J.H. (1989). Sexuality across the life course in the United States. In C.F. Turner, H.G. Miller and & L.E. Moses (Eds) *AIDS, Sexual Behaviour, and Intravenous Drug Use* (pp. 500–536). Washington, DC: National Academy Press.

Gagnon, J.H. and Simon, W. (1974) *Sexual Conduct: The social sources of human sexuality*. London: Hutchinson.

Gao, J.M. and Zhang, W. (1991) STD and population mobility: A China case study. *Chinese Social Medicine*, 36(5), 12–14.

Gil, V., Wang, S, Anderson, A. and & Lin, M. (1994) Plum blossoms and pheasants: Prostitutes, prostitution, and social control measures in contemporary China. *International Journal of Offender Therapy and Comparative Criminology*, 38(4), 319–337.

Gil, V., Wang, S., Anderson, A. and & Wu. L. (1996) Prostitutes, prostitution and STD/AIDS transmission in mainland China. *Social Science and Medicine*, 42(1), 141–152.

Guo, X.L. (1985) Behaviour issues and socioeconomic factors. *Journal of Chinese Juvenile Delinquency Research*, 6(3), 4–9.

Hearn, J. and Parkin, W. (1987) *Sex at Work: The power and paradox of organisation sexuality*. Brighton: Wheatsheaf Books.

Helman, C.G. (1990) *Culture, Health and Illness: An introduction for health professionals* (2nd edn). Oxford: Butterworth-Heinemann.

Herdt, G. and Abramson, P. R. (1990) The assessment of sexual practices relevant to the transmission of AIDS: A Global perspective. *The Journal of Sex research*, **27**(2), 215–232.

Herdt, G., Parker, R.G. and Carballo, M. (1991) HIV transmission, and AIDS research. *Journal of Sex Research*, 12(1), 78–88.

Herdt, G. and Stoller, R.J. (1990) *Intimate Communications*. New York: Columbia University Press.

Illsley. R. (1980) *Professional and Public Health: Sociology in health and medicine*. Nuffield Provincial Hospital Trust

Kippax, S., Crawford, J., Dowsett, G., Bond, G., Sinnott, V., Baxter, D., Berg, R., Connell, R. and Watson, L. (1990) Gay men's knowledge of HIV transmission and 'safe' sex: a question of accuracy. *Australian Journal of Social Issues*, 25(3), 199–219.

Kippax, S., Connell, R.W., Dowsett, G.W. and Crawford, J. (1993) *Sustaining Safe Sex: Gay communities respond to AIDS*. Lewes: The Falmer Press.

Kippax, S., Crawford, J., Connell, B., Dowsett, G., Watson, L., Rodden, P., Baxter, D. and Berg R. (1992) The importance of gay community in the prevention of HIV transmission: A study of Australian men who have sex with men, In P. Aggleton, P. Davies and G. Hart (Eds) *AIDS: Rights, risk and reason* (pp 103–118). Lewes: The Falmer Press.

Kuang, F.G. and Teng, C. (1989) Social and personal reasons about STD under-report: A survey on the under-report and not report for STD cases in private STD clinics. In Department of Anti-Epidemic and prevention of Minister of Public Health of China (Eds) *The Collected Papers for STD Preventive Work and Research Report*.

Ma, Y.G. (1990) *Sexology and its History*. Sichuan: Sichuan University Press.

MacLachlan, M. (1997) *Culture and Health*. Chichester: Wiley.

Malinowski, B. (1927). *Sex and Repression in Savage Society*. London: Routledge and Kegan Paul.

Malinowski, B. (1932) *The Sexual Life of Savages in North-western Melanesia* (3rd edn). London: Routledge and Kegan Paul.

Malinowski, B. (1960) *A Scientific Theory of Culture*. New York: Oxford University Press.

Manoff, S.B. (1989) Adolescence, AIDS epidemiology, prevention and public health (Z.P. Fan, Trans). *Chinese Journal of Epidemiology*, 21(4), 34–26.

McCamish, M. and Najman, J.M. (1995) AIDS and society. In G.M. Lupton and J.M. Najman (Eds) *Sociology of Health and Illness: Australian Readings*. University of Queensland Press.

Moore, S., Rosenthal, D. and Mitchell, A. (1996) *Youth, Aids and Sexually Transmitted Diseases*. London: Routledge.

National Centre for STD and AIDS Prevention of China (NCSAP), Ministry of Public Health (1997) Mainland China topics: HIV epidemic rapidly in China. *The Independence China Daily*, 21 November.

Orubuloye, I.O., Caldwell, J.C., Caldwell, P. and Santow, G. (1994) *Sexual Networking and AIDS in sub-Saharan Africa: Behavioural research and the social context*. Health Transition Centre, The Australian National University.

Parker, R.G., Herdt, G. and Carballo, M. (1991) Sexual culture, HIV transmission, and AIDS research. *The Journal of Sex Research*, 12(1), 77–78.

Pien, Y.J. (1989) Social structure and social control: the issues of prostitutes, prostitution and community control. *Social Journal of Sociology (China)*, 46(3), 7–11.

Pringle, R. (1988) *Secretaries Talk: Sexuality, power and work*. Sydney: Allen and Unwin.

Ruan, F.F. (1991) *Sex in China: Studies in sexology in Chinese culture*. New York: Plenum.

Rubin, G. (1975) The traffic in women: Notes on the 'political economy' of sex. In R. Reiter (Ed.) *Toward an Anthropology of Women*. New York: Monthly Review Press.

Scott, S. and Mercer, M. (1994) Understanding cultural obstacles to HIV/AIDS prevention in Africa. *AIDS Education & Prevention*, 6(1), 81–89.

Shiao, J.M. (1987) Prostitutes, prostitution and social control strategies. *Chinese Journal of Juvenile Delinquency Research*, 30(7), 16–25.

Shiao, J.M. (1992) A ten year study on prostitutes prostitution. *Chinese Journal of Juvenile Delinquency Research*, 95(9), 7–18.

Song, S. (1991) *Sexual Health and Practices in Ancient China*. Beijing: Chinese Medical Sciences and Techniques Publishing House.

Stevenson, E., Gertig, D., Crofts, N., Sherrard, J. and Breschkin, A. (1992) Three potential spectres of youth: chlamydia, gonorrhoea and HIV in Victorian youth. *Paper presented at the Australian Scientific Congress on Sexually Transmissible Diseases*, Sydney, November.

Wang, S. (1985) Chinese youth subcultural issues: a analysis of structure and function. *Society—Chinese Journal of Chinese Sociology*, 12, 11–15.

Wang, S. (1986a) *Youth Subculture and Hidden Movements in Society of China.* Guang Xi: Guang Xi Education and Science Publications.

Wang, S. (1986b) Sex, role and youth subculture. *Society—Chinese Journal of Sociology*, 12(2), 3–9.

Wang, S. (1987) Youth social behaviour and their social reference groups: A study on youth group's structure and function in urban China. *Chinese Journal of Youth Studies*, 42(3), 13–18.

Wang, S. (1989) *The Research on Juvenile Delinquency.* Sichuan: Sichuan Science and Technology Press.

Wang, S. (1998) *STD and AIDS-related risk-taking sexual behaviour within the dual employment system of Sichuan, China.* PhD thesis.

Wang, S., Gao, Y. and Zhao, J. W. (1998) Two cultures, two levels of AIDS risk. *World Health Forum (WHO)*, 19, 13–17.

Watney, S. (1990) Safe sex as community practice, In P. Aggleton, P. Daves and G. Hart (Eds) *AIDS: Individual, culture and policy dimensions.* Lewes: Falmer Press.

Williams, J.S. (1995) Theorising class, health and lifestyles: Can Bourdieu help us? *Sociology of Health and Illness—A Journal of Medical Sociology*, 17(5). 577–603.

Wuthnow, R., Hunter, J.D., Bergesen, A. and Kurzweil, E. (1990) *Cultural Analysis. USA.* London: Routledge & Kegan Paul (W.M. Li, Trans). Shanghai: Shanghai Runmei Chubanshe (Shanghai People's Publishing House) Press (original work published 1987).

Wu, J.L. and Wu C.G. (1982) Chinese collective behaviour: Insights from social psychology. *Paper given at the congress of Chinese association of social psychology on cross-cultural psychological studies.* YanJi, Jinlin, China. November.

Wu, J.L. and Wu, C.G. (1983) A study on collective behaviour: Behaviour test and change. *The Journal of Chinese Social Psychology*, 1(1), 3–10.

Xiao, G.H. (1993) China's labor market and employment of unemployed female workers. *Journal of Market Economic Research*, 32(2), 12–17.

Xu, W.Y. and Shao, C. (1996) A study on STD and HIV/AIDS epidemiology in China. In Department of anti-epidemic and prevention, Ministry of Public Health of China (Ed.) *The Collected Papers for STD Preventive Work and Research Report* (pp. 455–462). Beijing: Chinese Sciences and Technological Publications Press.

Xu, W. and Shao, C. (1997) STD epidemic and prevention-related issues. *Huaxi Jiankang Bao (West China Urban Public Health Weekly), 'STD/AIDS Prevention',* (8 December).

Yu, G.Y. (1989) Possession, ownership and their relationship to management. *Social Sciences of China*, 23(2), 3–23.

Zheng, X.W. (1997) Mainland China topics: China facing HIV epidemic: 200,000 HIV/AIDS cases had been reported in China. *The Independence Daily*, 3 December.

Chapter 5

Cultivating Health and the UN Convention on the Rights of the Child

Philip Cook

CASE STUDY

THE STORY OF JULIA (1980–1998)

Julia, who is 12 years old, lives with her family in the village of Chamulo, in the Mexican state of Quintana Roo. Julia is the youngest of four surviving children, and spends most of her day working in the maize field owned by her parents as part of the local *ejido* (communal land). Her family is very poor even by local standards. They live in substandard housing, and often do not have enough food to adequately feed all the children. Because of her family's need to include all the children in subsistence farming, Julia does not attend the local school. She often goes hungry, as the majority of the food is given to her brothers. Consequently, she has suffered from many childhood illnesses associated with malnutrition, and is undersized compared with other Mexican girls her age.

Julia's problems are compounded by her lack of Spanish, as she belongs to the predominantly Mayan population inhabiting Mexico's Yucatan peninsula. While this ethnic population forms the majority in the state in which Julia lives, they generally have less access to government services than the Spanish-speaking Ladino population. As a result, Julia not only does not participate in the local school but she also has not been properly immunized, nor has she received adequate preventive health education from government health-care workers.

Cultivating Health: Cultural Perspectives on Promoting Health. Edited by M. MacLachlan.
© 2001 John Wiley & Sons Ltd.

When Julia turns 13 her family decides she should go and work in the local city due to the declining price of corn caused by dwindling foreign markets for locally grown maize, since the advent of the North American Free Trade Agreement (NAFTA), and the need for additional revenue for the family. A neighbour has informed the family that work is available for Julia as a maid with a respectable Mexican family in a nearby city. Julia is connected with an agency that promises to provide her with such employment and a 'representative' from the agency picks her up from the village. Julia is taken to the city where she is told that the job with the family has fallen through and that she must instead work in a cheap restaurant serving tourists from Mexico and other Western countries.

Julia is now also informed that she owes the 'agency' US$300 for providing her with the job and allowing her to use a room in the back of the restaurant in which to sleep. Furthermore, Julia learns that many of the predominantly Mayan girls working in the restaurant are being forced to provide sexual favours to the guests to pay back their debt to the management.

Julia is soon also forced to engage in prostitution with customers in exchange for her room and board and to pay back the ever-increasing debt to the agency. She is severely beaten the one time she refuses to cooperate with her employer. After a number of years of physical abuse and sexual exploitation Julia notices that she is increasingly falling ill to minor illness, is losing weight and is becoming more easily fatigued. She now also has a young daughter, and needs to prostitute herself outside of the restaurant to pay for food and clothing for her child. One day she collapses at work and is taken by a colleague to a local clinic where she is eventually diagnosed as HIV positive.

Upon hearing that she has AIDS, her employer fires her and Julia and her daughter are forced to leave the restaurant and return to her village. Although her family is shunned by many of the other members of the village for the 'shame' their daughter has brought upon them, Julia is taken in by her family. There is no money for medicines to treat Julia's frequent and long-lasting infections. After a severe onset of illness Julia dies just prior to her eighteenth birthday.

INTRODUCTION

This case study highlights the vulnerability of children to certain situations placing them at high risk to disease, illness, and death. Such situations often hinge on issues of lack of basic rights, poor health promotion, and culture 'blind' and 'bound' services.

The health of children around the world remains a concern even with the bold promises for 'health for all by the year 2000' made at Alma Ata in 1978, and the broadening of the World Health Organization definition of health to encompass a 'state of complete physical and mental, and social well-being' and not merely 'the absence of disease and illness'. The current statistics clearly show the need to give serious and sustained attention to the health of children throughout the world, particularly in the less developed countries, but also in the so-called 'developed world'.

This chapter argues that children's health needs and the provision of basic health services must be more closely tied to a 'rights-based approach' in keeping with a broadening of the scope of children's health promotion resulting from the 1990 World Summit for Children and the subsequent global ratification of the United Nations Convention on the Rights of the Child (CRC). Such an approach represents a significant shift in the way children's health provision and promotion is conceived, for it forces societies to collectively assess the equity of health-care delivery and move beyond technology and disease-oriented responses to children's health, towards a more holistic understanding linking health and human rights. This in turn requires a broadening of the health debate to focus significant attention on the physical and social environment surrounding a child's development to include notions of family life, economic security, physical safety, community resources, civic vitality, and inter-sectoral partnership (Canadian Council on Social Development 1996). An understanding of the interplay between these variables and culture is critical in coming to grips with devising realistic strategies for implementing the child rights Convention at the local level.

According to the United Nations Children's Fund (UNICEF 1997) two thirds of under-5 deaths are caused by pneumonia, diarrhoea, measles, and malaria. Half of Asia's children are malnourished and in Africa one in three children is underweight (UNICEF 1998). Foetuses and children up to the age of three are most vulnerable to malnutrition. Roughly 35 000 children die in less developed countries each day, which on an annual basis equates to more than 12 million children. A new threat to children's health, in the form of HIV/AIDS, threatens to wipe out many of the gains made during the past twenty years in the form of children infected with the disease, and by eliminating many of the supports that children need most in the form of family, supportive community members, and health-care professionals themselves infected with HIV/AIDS.

Beyond a doubt, significant progress has been achieved during the last decade in protecting more children through immunization and greatly reducing the number of cases of polio, tetanus, and whooping cough. A great challenge still remains, however, in reaching the unreached, particularly the poorest and most marginalized children. Efforts must be made to strengthen the basis for sustained progress in improving health, through guaranteed basic health services, adequate nutrition, safe water, and sanitation, and family planning for these children and their families who continue to fall outside the coverage provided by existing health services. In addition, special protection measures need to be introduced to safeguard the security and healthy development of children at risk from political and social neglect, upheaval, and discrimination.

While the rate of child mortality and morbidity is currently much lower in the developed world, the progress achieved in reaching a relatively high rate of children's health in the industrialized world can no longer be taken as a given. The collapse of the Communist state health infrastructure in the

Eastern bloc countries and the subsequent jump in child morbidity rates, coupled with the increase in child poverty and homelessness in North America and associated health risks such as abuse, malnutrition, and reduced access to health care, provide clear evidence of the fragility of children's health promotion and prevention in industrialized nations (UNICEF 1998). Culture again becomes an important aspect of this threat to health equity in that many ethnic minorities and indigenous populations experience various forms of discrimination in accessing health-care services.

A number of recent developments have provided new approaches and opportunities to address the global inequalities in children's health. These include: the international development of child health goals established at the World Summit for Children and resulting Plan of Action; subsequent international summits for social action such as the World Summit for Social Development; and the near-universal ratification of the Convention on the Rights of the Child. When taken as a whole these frameworks provide an ecology, or socially supportive system, of children's rights to survival and healthy development.

Finally, there is growing support for a population health approach to children's well-being that seeks to address the social determinants of health, specifically examining why some people are healthier than others, before suggesting how available resources should be determined and distributed to maximize the health status of the total population. In Canada, and a number of developing nations this approach is being seriously considered by local and national governments and other sectors of civil society, with the result that there is now a greater focus on strategic childhood health interventions to deepen the impact over a persons entire life span.

THE WORLD SUMMIT FOR CHILDREN, DECLARATION AND PLAN OF ACTION

The World Summit for Children, which took place in September 1990, resulted in a number of goals for children in the 1990s and established health targets for the year 2000. These goals have provided clear and measurable progress for improving children's well-being including malnutrition, preventable disease, and illiteracy. Of equal importance has been the unparalleled success in creating an enabling environment to implement these goals through a global advocacy process supported by United Nations agencies, governments, non-governmental organizations (NGOs), and community members.

The Summit goals, outlined in the World Declaration and Plan of Action on the Survival, Protection, and Development of Children (UNICEF 1991), include targeted reductions in infant and maternal mortality, child malnutrition and illiteracy, as well as improved levels of access to basic services for health and family planning, education, water, and sanitation. Specific decade goals were set for the year 2000, and intermediate goals were established for 1995.

Within three years of the Summit, 105 industrialized and developing nations, covering a total of 88% of the world's children had prepared national programmes of action (NPAs) for meeting the World Summit goals.

These goals represent a significant global commitment to improve children's basic survival and development requirements. A major focus is placed on children's health and education, with an emphasis on early intervention strategies to reduce early childhood morbidity and mortality.

The 10th Summit goal addresses child protection issues through the target of achieving universal ratification of the Convention on the Rights of the Child, including improved protection for children in especially difficult circumstances. However, the major Summit success lies in its setting specific and measurable primary health and education goals, and in creating a framework through the national programmes of action, to mobilize resources to achieve these goals.

Thus far, the Mid Decade goals have been largely successfully met. In fact, UNICEF estimates that due to countries success in implementing the Decade goals roughly three quarters of a million fewer children each year will be blinded, crippled, or mentally retarded (UNICEF 1996). Particular success stories include the eradication of polio in the Western Hemisphere and the significant reduction of polio in East Asia and the Middle East and North Africa, as well as the reduction in childhood blindness caused by vitamin A deficiency, and the retreat of measles.

In order that resources be shared more equitably for children in countries with fewer resources, industrialized nations are asked to increase levels of aid to less developed countries to 0.7% of their GNP. ODA specifically targets humanitarian and development purposes, from which military aid is excluded. About two thirds of ODA is bilateral, and is donated directly from one government to another. The remaining third is multilateral, and is directed via international organizations, NGOs, and United Nations agencies. Currently, counter to popular beliefs, ODA levels fall far short of this goal, at approximately 0.3%. Only a quarter of this goes to the 50 least developed nations: less than one sixth goes to agriculture and even less ends up in the social sector (UNICEF 1998). This situation continues to worsen with the demise of many former Eastern bloc economies resulting in a large reduction of aid from this sector of the industrialized world to less developed countries.

A recent strategy to help raise and better direct ODA is the 20/20 formula. The 20/20 strategy was introduced by Norway and launched at the World Summit for Social Development in Copenhagen in 1995. The formula suggests an allocation of 20% of the recipient governments' national budget and 20% of the donor countries' AIDs budget to basic social services. The 20/20 formula has been jointly adopted by the UNDP, UNESCO, UNICEF, and WHO. If accepted, this proposed strategy could have a significant impact in reaching societies' poorest and most vulnerable, in particular children.

While the World Summit for children has been undeniably successful, some of the Summit goals have been more difficult to achieve, most notably the reduction of maternal mortality (UNICEF 1996). Increasingly, the realization of Health for All is being tied to programmes targeting poverty and resource reallocation. Similarly, the more difficult goal of supporting children in especially difficult circumstances will likely never be reached unless the fundamental problem of social and economic marginalization of the poorest nations and the poorest people, including children and youth, is addressed. The primary obstacle to achieving adequate health care and education is poverty—a barrier both against contributing to or benefiting from the processes of economic and social development.

This was acknowledged globally in the Copenhagen Summit goals of 1995 which specifically attempt to address issues relating to the distribution of economic growth, discrimination against women and children, particularly girls, and the deterioration of the environment. The three broad objectives underlining the Copenhagen Summit include: the reduction of the proportion of people living in absolute poverty; the creation of the necessary jobs and sustainable livelihoods; and the significant reduction in disparities among various income classes, sexes, age groups, ethnic groups, geographical regions, and nations. For children, these goals reflect a broadening of focus from basic child survival and development mirrored in the Children's Summit goals to more widespread social reform. The challenge of the next decade will be to apply the ingredients for success from the Children's Summit goals and implementing mechanisms and apply them to the deeper and more challenging social issues impacting on children's health.

Richard Jolly, former UNICEF Deputy Executive Director for Programmes at UNICEF, describe these expanded Children's Summit strategies as follows (UNICEF 1995):

> 'This mixture—which I term a new paradigm for development action—is I believe of widespread applicability. Just as the success of immunization over the 1980s has led to a broader agenda of goals for improving the health and welfare of children, so this model could also be applied to other areas of international action; to new approaches to peacemaking and conflict prevention; to human development focused on the eradication of poverty; to strengthening of human rights and democratic processes; to environmental protection and sustainable development; to managing of global economic and financial relationships.' (p. 41)

The Convention on the Rights of the Child, in protecting all the rights of children and not only those targeted in the World Summit goals, allows for an holistic approach to promoting the well-being of all children in both developing and developed nations. It provides, for the first time, a language supporting children's well-being that is global. All children now have human rights, and while the specific issues facing a child in Cambodia may differ from a child in Great Britain their civil, political, social, economic, and cultural rights are the same.

A 'RIGHTS' APPROACH TO CHILDREN'S HEALTH

The Children's Convention, adopted by the UN General Assembly in 1989, and entered into force on 2 September, 1990, has now become a human rights landmark by reaching near-universal ratification in record time. As of

June 1998, it has been ratified by 191 out of 193 nation states. Only Somalia, which at that time had no government, and the United States, which has signed and has yet to ratify, remain outside of nations bound by the Convention. In its preamble and 54 articles, the children's Convention provides a comprehensive paradigm for supporting the totality of children's healthy development, drawing on the support of governments and non-governmental organizations alike, and is revolutionary in promoting children's participation in reaching minimum standards of care and protection including those of health care, education, and child protection.

The Convention on the Rights of the Child (CRC) for the first time recognizes the child as a full human being with his or her own unique identity distinct from that of their parents and community. The Convention follows in the footsteps of the Universal Declaration of Human Rights, and the Covenants on Civil and Political Rights and Economic, Social, and Cultural Rights. The CRC establishes social and economic rights for children—the right to survival and early development, education, health care and social assistance. It also covers civil and political rights. These include the right of a child to a name and a nationality, to freedom of expression, to participation in decisions affecting his or her well-being. and to protection from discrimination on the grounds of race, gender, or minority status, as well as protection from sexual and other forms of abuse and exploitation.

Countries ratifying the CRC must submit periodic reports to a committee of ten experts making up the UN Committee on the rights of the Child. In these reports, governments must report on the steps taken to change national laws and formulate policies and programmes supporting children's rights. UNICEF and non-governmental organizations play an important role in helping the Committee assess the accuracy and completeness of country reports through the submission of alternative reports and supplementary information.

Article 24 of the Convention is devoted to the health rights of the child. It builds on and develops the right to life, survival and development as set out in article 6. The key provisions of article 24 reflect a broad-based definition of health with the overall goal of reducing infant and child mortality through 'the enjoyment of the highest attainable standard of health'.

Specific actions are also laid out to address health promotion and prevention through the principles of primary health care, specifically by combining health knowledge with social action on specific goals (i.e. basic knowledge of child health and nutrition, promoting breast-feeding, hygiene, and environmental sanitation). Article 24 also targets the right of the child to protection from traditional practices prejudicial to the health of the child. Finally, article 24 encourages countries to undertake international cooperation in promoting children's health, especially in developing countries.

Other articles in the CRC that complement article 24 are: article 2 (non-discrimination); article 23 (rights of a child with a disability); articles 26 (the right to social assistance) and 27 (right to an adequate standard of living); and articles 28 (right to education) and 29 (the aims of education). Article 24 thus holistically links the promotion of child health to equity and the role of the state in ensuring social support and assistance. It also suggests a close relationship between a child's health and 'the development of the child's personality, talents and mental and physical abilities to their full potential' (article 29.1.a).

The Committee on the Rights of the Child places significant emphasis on article 24 in country reports. State parties are requested to provide information including: the status and indicators of children's health (i.e. incidence of HIV/AIDS): current legislation and responsible agencies; distribution of services (i.e. rural/urban); persistent gaps and measures adopted to reduce existing disparities; prevalence of educational campaigns; as well as specific information on women and children's health.

While the reporting process has been constructive and has resulted in significant and important improvements for children's health, problems remain. Some countries have been very progressive in addressing the reporting guidelines on health. For example, Panama's initial report discussed the disproportional high incidence of disease amongst indigenous children (Panama, Initial Report, paras 153 and 155). Many countries, however, have missed their reporting deadlines, and implementing the CRC beyond ratification is still in its infancy.

One of the conceptual tensions being played out in the debate on international children's health is the discussion about 'basic needs' and 'basic services' and the rift between 'human rights' specialists and 'human development'. Parker and Sepulveda (1995) rightly describe both philosophical approaches as 'tilling the same land'. The fundamental difference lies in the human development community emphasizing the need to position the technologies and services needed to provide 'basic services' to satisfy the 'basic needs' of the population. The human rights community instead focuses on identifying and developing legal instruments and the enforcement mechanisms needed to support human development activities (Parker and Sepulveda 1995). Indeed, one of the aims of a rights approach is to build on the success of the technological advances of child health made during the last 20 years, for example, immunization programmes. This offers a much-needed avenue for furthering the success of the Summit and goals in order to more effectively and ethically addresses issues of equity with regard to economic and social mobilization for all children irrespective of a child's gender, race or minority status, and age.

PROMOTING AN 'ECOLOGY' OF CHILDREN'S WELL-BEING: COMBINING PERSPECTIVES OF POPULATION HEALTH, DETERMINANTS OF HEALTH AND CHILDREN'S RIGHTS

The CRC can help strengthen the links between social policy and health policy when combined with other health-promotion paradigms. Two such paradigms are the population health approach and determinants of health:

'A population health approach examines the collective health of individuals, studying while some individuals are healthier than others, why the differences are systematically spread across discernible social gradients, and how public resources are most effectively deployed.' (Hayes 1994: 1)

'Determinants of health' comprise a set of significant health factors that influence the health of children and adults. A growing body of research indicates key determinants for children's healthy development include factors such as: income and social status; social support and networks; education; employment and working conditions; social environments; physical environments; biological and genetic inheritance; health services; gender; and culture (Canadian Department of Health 1997). Both frameworks are collective, as opposed to individualistic and comprise a broad-based approach to health as opposed to equating health with the availability of health care. They are therefore compatible with the interpretation of children's health rights thus far discussed in this chapter.

This theoretical synthesis has two positive outcomes. First, principles of population health targeting children grounded in research on determinants of children's health can help guide strategic implementation of children's rights. Second, a rights approach can provide an ethical and legal framework for health policy. Primary foundations from both perspectives include:

(1) The key determinants of children's health
    The social and economic environment
    The physical environment
    Personal health practices
    Individual capacity and coping skills
    And existing health services.
(2) The four 'pillars' of the CRC:
    Non-discrimination (CRC article 2)
    Best interests (CRC article 3)
    Life, survival and development (CRC article 6) and participation (CRC article 12).

When combined they become a powerful advocacy model of an 'ecology' for children's health. Such an 'ecology' of health refers to the 'systems' of support required by a child to develop to the maximum of his or her abilities.

This notion builds on Uri Bonfenbrenner's (1979, 1990) theory of the social ecology of human development. In this framework, Bronfenbrenner places the child at the centre of a series of socially nested systems. This begins with the mesosystem, or those people immediately in contact with the child (family, peers, teachers, other caretakers etc.), and continuing out to the macrosystem or wider society and socio-cultural norms and values of the child's social environment. Bronfenbrenner (1990) argues that all systems need to be mutually supportive for optimal healthy development to occur.

The effective functioning of child rearing processes in the family and other child settings requires public policies and practices that provide place, time, stability, status, recognition, belief systems, customs and actions in support of child-rearing activities not only on the parts of the parents, caregivers, teachers and other professional personnel, but also relatives, friends, neighbours, co-workers, communities and major economic, social and political institutions of the entire society (Bonfenbrenner 1990: 9).

The social ecology of child development provides a theory for children's well-being that establishes a common ground for both the comprehensive social ethic of a child rights approach and the population approach to children's health determinants. This then becomes a framework for establishing an empirical and moral minimum for children's development.

While the specific issues affecting children in developing countries and in industrial nations may differ in character (e.g. maternal and child survival, and provision of basic services versus services for child abuse or teenage pregnancy), such a framework provides a common ground for promoting a 'First Call' so that children's rights and well-being be given precedence especially in times of economic hardship. Areas for research based on an ecology of children's rights would require an examination of certain areas where family, community, or socio-cultural support of the child is not functioning or under pressure from external forces. Examples might include, social breakdown due to rapid economic change, and lack of an integrated child focused policy at the local, national or international level.

When examining the gaps in the current global social ecology of children's healthy development some specific areas for research and programme development emerge. These would include first, better understanding children and childhood. If health researchers and children's advocates are serious about children's well being and child rights, then greater attention needs to be focused on understanding children's lives and the ways in which childhood is constructed in various social settings. As Qvortrup (1993) explains, childhood is a framework for the organization and the location of the various social spaces in which children participate and through which they pass. Childhood is therefore a 'permanent social category', that shows variation across time and cultural context.

The Convention is itself a framework based on certain concepts of childhood promoting the right of a child to a quality of life during this time of a person's life. For example, the preamble to the CRC describes childhood as a human condition during which the individual is entitled to 'special care and assistance'. Furthermore, article 1 defines childhood as every human being below the age of eighteen years (the rights of the foetus are not specifically addressed in the Convention).

Knutson (1997), in his book *Children: Noble citizens or worthy causes*, eloquently describes the importance of better understanding the various social perspectives on childhood (including children's own perceptions of their lives). This is especially important in order to untangle the rhetoric of a 'child-saving' society based on uninformed and arbitrary notions of welfare, from a society whose social attitudes are more oriented towards notions of 'children first' and a rights approach.

Research building on the work of Qvortrup and others (Qvortrup *et al.* 1990; Knutson 1997; Qvortrup 1993) is needed to better understand how social policy promoting children's health development is itself based on unacknowledged assumptions regarding the role of children in society and the value placed on childhood.

Second, research is needed to deconstruct economic security and children's rights. As discussed, in both the developing and developed world great gains have been made in child survival. The greatest challenge in both contexts is to address the right to a healthy development for children falling between the cracks of current economic policy and service programming.

In addressing the needs of economic equity for children, the Convention through the lens of article 2 (non-discrimination) provides guidelines for the equitable distribution of resources in two other articles. These are articles 4 (implementation of the Convention) targeting general measures of implementation, including appropriate legislative administrative measures; participation of civil society; and international cooperation), and 27 (child's right to an adequate standard of living) including a standard of living adequate for physical, mental, spiritual, moral and social development; parent's primary responsibility, states duty to support the child and family qualified by national conditions and means; nutrition and housing; and the child's rights to maintenance.

Confronting issues of economic, social and political discrimination of groups of children is a critical area of advocacy for children's equitable health. Population health research has shown that in regions where the gaps between rich and poor are large the health discrepancies between these groups is disproportionately large. Mothers and children from lower socioeconomic groups are thus at higher risk than other sectors of the population to low birth weight, chronic health problems, and premature death (Avard 1994).

Children and youth who are marginalized from the wider civil society, including: children living in poverty, girls, street children, children who are sexually exploited, and children from certain ethnic minorities and aboriginal children are also more prone to injury and illness than other sectors of society with greater access to resources and information (Canadian Council on Social Development 1996). Child-protection strategies therefore need to be better understood within the context of social and cultural marginalization and economic disparity. The CRC places considerable emphasis on the issue of non-discrimination and importance of children's cultural rights. The preamble to the Convention sets the tone for the following articles by underscoring 'the importance of the traditions and cultural values of each people for the protection and harmonious development of the child'.

Social marginalization and cultural are important mitigating factors in the health of children of ethnic minorities and indigenous children. Specific articles in the Convention addressing cultural and minority rights include: article 2 (non-discrimination); article 4 (provision of resources to support cultural rights); article 5 (respect for family of child as provided by local cultures); article 14 (freedom of thought, conscience and religion); article 20 (respect of culture of orphaned child); article 29 (need for education respecting culture); article 30 (respect for the cultural rights of indigenous and minority children); and article 31 (right to participate in cultural and artistic life).

Two issues are paramount in examining the rights of children from minority cultures to basic services, the right to equality and the right to diversity. For these children, accessibility to health services depends on such things as: economic accessibility (ability to access services due to lack of material resources); physical accessibility (distance from family and community-many minority children live in remote locations); linguistic accessibility (providing services in local languages); and cultural accessibility (ensuring services respect and support local values and beliefs).

Accessibility to adequate health care for minority and indigenous peoples generally suffers a deficit of these factors. In addition, the health status of these children is difficult to measure due to a lack of accurate statistics, and greater disaggregation of available data is needed in this area. However, where data is available, trends point to poorer health status. For example, a recent Royal Commission on Aboriginal peoples in Canada revealed that, on average, an indigenous child in Canada is more likely to suffer from a preventable birth defect, become injured as a child, contract HIV/AIDS, and commit suicide than his non-native peers. Similarly, recent statistics gathered by UNICEF Mexico indicate that children living in Mexican states with high numbers of indigenous peoples (e.g. Chiapas, Oaxaca) have significantly less access to basic services and experience chronic shortage of water and malnutrition in comparison to Mexican states with low numbers of indigenous peoples. In Latin America, a disturbing trend is emerging in which increasing numbers of minority and indigenous children are engaged in economic migration. This results in even greater vulnerability of these children as they are removed from the protective mechanisms of their communities, and are exposed to potentially dangerous working conditions, and various forms of exploitation and abuse.

Finally, research is needed that seeks to better understand the impact of social and physical environmental factors on children. One of the key findings in the research on the health determinants is that the social environment in which children live, from conception through early adulthood, has long-lasting effects over their entire life span. Mustard and Frank (1991) point out that how children are cared for at an early age can influence their coping skills for the rest of their lives.

Keating and Mustard (1993) similarly note the strong evidence of the relationship between development of competency and coping skills, the social context of everyday life, and individual health and well-being, and the relationship between growth prosperity, social environment and individual development. The focus on children's perceptions of their lives supports the growing literature on children's coping styles and resiliency (Fraser 1997; Werner and Smith 1992). An important question for policy makers and human service practitioners is what kind of intervention may help individuals overcome barriers to health development set in early life. One of the characteristics of high-risk children who do well despite the odds is that they were able to find at least one significant person who cared about them in the community in which they live (Goulet 1994).

This kind of buffering notion is supported in the Convention's focus on respect and support for the rights of the parents, extended family, and community in article 5. Similarly, article 18 supports the responsibilities of parents for children's well-being, with the best interests of the child being their primary concern. Article 18 also acknowledges the importance of day care as a buffering factor for children of working parents.

Keating and Mustard (1993) also discuss the health impact of the physical environment. The authors cite research findings from Eastern Europe where following initial improvements in their economies and their health after the Second World War both their economies and health status of their populations have declined over the last 2 years. In some cases, the authors argue, particularly in countries like Poland, that this decline is contemporaneous with industrial pollution. This problem is not confined solely to heavily industrialized countries, as recent research, particularly in the circumpolar countries, is showing the effect that environmental pollutants are having in neighbouring regions linked by common weather patterns and ocean currents.

The importance of the environment is critical to a child's life, survival, and health development (article 6). There is also a growing realization that children's psycho-social well-being is partially related to a sense of interconnectedness with their environment. This relationship, while difficult to prove quantitatively, is becoming more apparent in studies linking indigenous children's health to self identity in terms of a personal sense of connectedness with traditional indigenous lands and knowledge of their tribal language (ECOSOC 1996; Pepper and Henry 1992). In this regard, it is important to find ways of linking the various international treaties that speak to children's health and the environment. The most important of these treaties is the Rio Declaration on the Environment and Development (including Agenda 21) ratified in 1992. The Rio Declaration emphasizes the need to educate children on the need for sustainable development and care for the natural environment. Specifically, Principle 10 states: 'Environmental issues are best handled with the concerns of all concerned citizens, at the relevant level'. Principle 21 strengthens the role of youth in this process by stating 'the creativity, ideals, and courage of the youth of the world should be mobilized to forge a global partnership in order to achieve sustainable development for all'. In implementing an ecology of children's rights to health, Hodgekin and Newell (1998) suggest a number of measures. These fall under categories of general measures of implementation and specific measures in implementing article 24.

First, with regard to general measures, responsible departments and agencies for children's health should be identified at all levels of government. Similarly, non-governmental agencies and civil society partners should be identified. Other general measures include: a review of the relevant legislation, policy and practice; the adoption of a strategy to secure full implementation including rights-based indicators and relevant standards;

making the implications of article 24 widely known to adults and children; and development of appropriate training of all relevant human service professionals involved in children's health.

Specific monitoring measures suggested by the authors include: identifying the degree to which the state has implemented article 24 to the maximum extent of available resources; promoting the participation and views of the child in decisions affecting him or her (e.g. planning and developing health care and decision making in relation to individual health treatment of the child); assessing the accessibility and quality of services for children with a disability, girls and other marginalized children; measuring success or failure in attaining the World Summit goals for health; and identifying the degree to which the state supports social and environmental health through health education, health promotion, and support to public health especially for parents and children (Hodgekin and Newell 1998).

These provide a useful assessment tool for measuring state support for children's health that include perspectives of rights and population health. They also provide a starting place for moving from implementation of rights through ratification of the CRC setting goals and developing health strategies for children that build on global initiatives such as the World Summit and are supported by research on determinants of children's health.

This success of combining these perspectives will be measured by the commitment of governments and civil society to heed the growing knowledge on the determinants of children's healthy development while simultaneously promoting social equity based on a respect for children as full and equal members of society.

CONCLUSION

Implications stemming from the adoption of a 'rights-based' approach to children's health promotion call for responses at various social and political levels. Returning to the case study at the beginning of the chapter, we can see that Julia's health is compromised from the moment she is born by belonging to a sector of the population (in this case the indigenous Mayas) that experiences a high degree of discrimination.

The resulting social marginalization caused by this discrimination leads to her falling between the cracks of appropriate medical coverage in both health prevention (proper immunization) and promotion (culturally appropriate health education). Discrimination also impacts her prospects for healthy life, survival and development through her lack of nutrition, inability to attend school, and the subsequent need for her to seek employment outside of the potentially protective mechanisms of her family, community, and culture.

Similarly, Julia's best interests, and those of countless children like her, are generally not taken into consideration when trade agreements like NAFTA are drafted and ratified, thus leading to the further economic and social marginalization of vulnerable sectors of the population, especially women and children.

Finally, Julia is placed at greater risk of suffering from various types of abuse, such as sexual exploitation, and of contracting diseases like HIV/ AIDS. Such diseases discriminate in favour of girls like Julia due to her economic and educational poverty and an accompanying lack of power associated with this poverty. She is at greater risk of having her health and well-being compromised by the impact of global tourism, as this can have a particularly negative affect on vulnerable children and women living in communities undergoing rapid social and economic upheaval.

Rights-based strategies aimed at improving the health of children like Julia must start with the ratification of the CRC. This then leads to the need to assess existing laws and social policy affecting children and their families through the lens of the Convention. National Plans of Action based on the Summit Goals of children's rights to health care, education, and social protection need to be developed. Universal and appropriate coverage of all of the Summit goals may be challenging for poor countries without adequate resources. In this case, there is a need for developed nations to bring their ODA in line with the Convention by allocating appropriate and sufficient support to international development programmes benefiting children and their families living in especially difficult circumstances.

Education is particularly important in fostering positive attitudes towards the rights of all children and their families, especially disadvantaged and marginalized sectors of society. This also entails identifying cultural values and beliefs supporting the rights of the child, and challenging attitudes and stereotypes that are harmful to children.

Finally, and perhaps most importantly, children's voices need to be heard and considered in debates both at the local and national level in determining health priorities as well as in shaping delivery modalities that can be best integrated into the lives of children. This means providing children with age-appropriate information to make informed decisions and opportunities to safely practise these rights with guidance from their elders. It also means consulting with children's parents and supporting the rights of families to raise their children in the spirit of 'peace, dignity, tolerance, freedom, and understanding'.

Reaching these goals will not be achieved easily or quickly. However, applying a rights perspective to children's health promotion may help shift the momentum of universal health coverage further from a history of health care as charity and closer to health as an inalienable part of every individual's healthy human development.

REFERENCES

Avard, D. (1994) Poverty and child health. Ottawa: Human Rights and Education Centre. Unpublished report.

Bronfenbrenner, U. (1979) *The Ecology of Human Development: Experiments by nature and design.* Cambridge, MA: Harvard University Press.

Bronfenbrenner, U. (1990) Discovering what families do. In D. Blankenhorn, D. Bayme and J.B. Elshtain (Eds) *Rebuilding the Nest: A new commitment to the American family*. Milwaukee, WI: Family Service America.

Canadian Council on Social Development (CCSD) (1996) *The Progress of Canada's Children 1996*. Ottawa: CCSD.

Canadian Department of Health (1997) Towards a common understanding: Clarifying the core concepts of population health. A discusssion paper. Ottawa: Government of Canada.

Economic and Social Council (ECOSOC) (1996) *Health and Indigenous Peoples*. 11 June. Geneva: ECOSOC.

Fraser, M. (1997) *Risk and Resilience in Childhood: An ecological perspective*. Washington, DC: NASW Press.

Goulet, L. (1994) The UN Convention on the Rights of the Child: Giving voice. University of Victoria: Unpublished curriculum.

Hayes, M., Foster, L.T. and Foster, H.D. (1994) *The Determinants of Population Health: A critical assessment*. Victoria, BC: Western Geographical Series, Vol. 29.

Hodgekin, R. and Newell, P. (1998) *Implementation Handbook for the Convention on the Rights of the Child*. New York: UNICEF.

Keating, D. and Mustard, F. (1993) *Social Economic Factors and Human Devlopment*. Ottawa: CCSD.

Knutson, E. (1997) *Children: Noble Causes or Worthy Citizens*. Aldershot: Arena.

Mustard, F. and Frank, I. (1991) *The Determinants of Health*. Canadian Institute for Advanced Research, Publication 5.

Parker, D. and Sepulveda, C. (1995) Children's rights to survival and healthy development. In J. Himes (Ed.) *Implementing the Convention on the Rights of the Child: Resource mobilization in low-income countries*. The Hague: Martinus Nijhoff.

Pepper, F. and Henry, S. (1992) *An Indian Perspective on Self-esteem*. Vancouver BC: Mowachat Education and Research Association.

Qvortrup, J. (1993) Childhood as a social phenomenon: Lessons from an international project. Eurosocial reports, 47, Vienna: European Centre for Social Welfare Policy and Research.

Qvortrup, J., Bardy, M., Sgritta, G. and Wintersberger, H. (Eds) *Childhood Matters: Social theory, practice, and politics*. Aldershot: Avebury.

United Nations Children's Fund (UNICEF) (1991) *The World Summit for Children: The World Declaration and Plan of Action*. New York: United Nations Children's Fund.

UNICEF (1995) *The State of the World's Children 1995*. New York: UNICEF.

UNICEF (1996) *The State of the World's Children 1996*. New York: UNICEF.

UNICEF (1998) *The State of the World's Children 1998*. New York: UNICEF.

Werner, E. and Smith, R. (1992) *Overcoming the Odds: High risk children from birth to adulthood*. Ithaca, NY: Cornell University Press.

Part II
PLURALISM AND CULTIVATING HEALTH

Chapter 6

Asian Psychological Approaches and Western Therapy

Dan Berkow and Richard C. Page

For the past half-century, there has been a growing influence of Asian psychological approaches on the practice of Western therapy. This influence has occurred as Western theorists and practitioners have attempted to enlarge and clarify their awareness of the person, especially regarding the promotion, maintenance, and re-establishment of wholeness for persons struggling with disease or problematic patterns in living and relating. Western therapy continues to draw on models of the person and reality that have evolved over centuries of cultural development that has included science, art, ethics, and history as important factors. However, many Western thinkers and practitioners have integrated ideas and practices from Asian psychologies as they addressed concerns that could not be fully encompassed within a strictly Western frame of reference. Among a multitude of possible examples are such influential therapists and theorists as Maslow (1971), Epstein (1995), Goleman (1976, 1981), Jung (1964), Murphy and Murphy (1968), Perls (1972), and Rogers (1980).

The influence of Asian psychology has not been limited to the theory and practice of therapy. Ideas from Asian psychology influenced Western culture through Zen Buddhist ideas that affected the 'Beat Generation' of poets, writers and philosophers including Ginsberg (1959), Kerouac (1958), and Ferlinghetti (1958). Additionally, T'ai Ch'i has become a popular mode of exercise in the West, Asian martial arts are available for study in most Western cities and towns, and books on topics such as herbology or meditation and health are commonplace. The diaspora of Tibetan Buddhists from

Cultivating Health: Cultural Perspectives on Promoting Health. Edited by M. MacLachlan.
© 2001 John Wiley & Sons Ltd.

an occupied country has led to greater dissemination of once hidden teachings of Tibetan Buddhism, and the Dalai Lama (1997) has written books, spoken to many Western audiences and has been the subject of two major motion pictures. Cultural exchange occurs in many directions, and we can find many examples of Western beliefs and practices that have influenced Asian therapies and health care. For example, Morita therapy incorporates ideas from Western psychology with concepts from Zen Buddhism (Reynolds 1984).

Successful integration of Western and Eastern ideas of healing will require: being respectful of one's own culture and healing practices, not overvaluing or treating as final answers the input from another culture that seems 'mysterious' or 'mystical', being aware of how to work within one's culture in terms of communication and action while using ideas from outside that culture in appropriate ways, and enlarging and deepening one's view of self and reality to form a more inclusive picture while respecting differences between concepts from different cultures. As we work on forming a more comprehensive view, we need to question biases that may limit the scope of our awareness and practice. Successful integration requires not simply adding new ideas to old but transforming the old perspective to allow the new one to function successfully. In other words, forming a new and more comprehensive gestalt (i.e. meaning-whole) involves letting go of assumptions and beliefs that artificially limit and constrain the emerging new meaning.

The old ideas in Western philosophy and psychology that oppose logic to intuition and body to mind (or which try to eliminate mind and replace it with chemical interactions) give way to a new view in which logic works with intuition, in which awareness can include yet work outside of logical categories, and in which mind and body can inform each other in a unitive manner without doing away with the importance of either. A dualistic framework gives way to a new non-dualistic integration. Asian psychologies have differed in the language and symbolism they used, yet consistently found ways to express that 'the way things are' does not involve any ultimate opposition of forces, or any ultimately separable categories into which reality can be divided.

The case of Karen, which is presented in this chapter, illustrates how thinking from a non-dualistic framework, such as is emphasized in Asian psychologies, can be applied to counseling. A study of theorists who have written about the value of a perspective beyond dualism in philosophy and psychology (e.g. Chan 1963; Goleman 1981; Watts 1966, 1972; Welwood 1996; Wilber 1980) indicates that certain themes lend themselves to using a nondualistic perspective in therapeutic or healing work. The following themes are consistently presented in important writings and research on Asian psychologies: (1) valuing compassion, (2) non-imposition of perspectives, (3) appreciation of balance as linked to health, (4) 'letting go' as a means to effect growth, (5) releasing faulty assumptions about the self, (6) attention and awareness considered as inherently valuable, (7) change considered as a basic and continuous reality, (8) the harmonized flow of energy as intrinsic to life and well-being, (9) spiritual development as intrinsic to personal and social development, and (10) reliance on intution as well as logic. These ten themes are unitive of Asian psychologies in the sense that, although many important variations can be found in Asian perspectives concerning the person and well-being, these themes are similarly valued in several key Asian approaches. Hinduism, Buddhism, and Taoism, in particular, have addressed each of these themes (e.g. see Chan 1963, Watts 1972). We have selected these ten themes as key areas in which Western psychological approaches can integrate concepts from Asian psychological approaches.

In this chapter, we will see that Karen's therapy used these principles, and that such principles can be usefully applied to working with a variety of clients in counseling and therapy—to 'wellness' concerns, that is, to promotion of well-being as well as remediation of distress. We note that in discussing this case we have used the words 'counseling' and 'therapy' as relatively interchangeable, as the overlapping areas of meaning in these two concepts seem to us to outweigh the differences. Although therapy is often treated as more in-depth work than counseling, and focusing more on insight than support, we have found that depth of focus frequently shifts, and support and insight are far from mutually exclusive therapeutic modes.

CASE STUDY

KAREN

Karen was a student with whom one of the authors worked in counseling. She attended a university full-time and worked part-time at a local movie theatre. Karen enjoyed athletics, was in generally good health, maintained consistent eye contact during interactions, and had an engaging smile. During the beginning phase of counseling, however, smiles were rare—Karen came across as preoccupied, tense and anxious. Toward the end of counseling, Karen presented as visibly more relaxed, with a sense of humor that could be either playful or sarcastic, and a more engaged way of interacting.

In her initial session, Karen described multiple interacting areas of difficulty. Problem areas included persistent anxiety and tension around academic and social concerns, dependence on alcohol, frequent use of marijuana, persistent depressive symptoms, and lack of confidence about her future and her relationships. In our fourth session, she disclosed uncertainty about her sexual orientation. Worries about herself, and the ways that others saw her, frequently arose at night and often interfered with her sleep. She reported symptoms of dysthymia, or long-term low-level depression. These included feelings of emptiness and futility on a daily basis, generally low levels of energy, a tendency to mentally 'drift off' when she needed to focus, and an apathetic reaction to work, school, and friends. At times, lack of sleep and low energy became associated with intense self-negativity and feelings of hopelessness about her life and her future. She would eat little food during these periods but would still manage to get to class, go through the motions at work, and get her homework done. Usually after a few days of reduced food intake, she would begin to eat more and thus gain energy to an extent.

Karen's stated philosophy was 'I have to believe in myself no matter what, and I have to believe I can get where I want to go in life'. For her, this meant being able to help others who might have fewer financial or educational advantages than she had. Karen frequently complained about experiences of physical tension, especially in her lower abdomen. She had bouts of colitis that had led to hospitalization about two years ago. Asthma was a problem when she was younger, but had receded with adulthood.

Karen was a white graduate student in her mid-twenties majoring in Education. She was generally physically healthy, wore her brown hair long, and tended to dress informally but appropriately. She could have moments of vibrant connection, but usually portrayed a listless and rather disengaged persona. She was raised in a small farming community close to a Midwestern American city. Her parents tried to instill what they considered to be 'good Christian values'. Karen had powerful ambivalent feelings toward her parents, seeing them as loving her in a way she could not clearly understand. Their love seemed to be expressed in their physical presence and willingness to 'provide' for her in a material way. She perceived them as unable to express affection toward each other or her. Her father strove to work hard and suppress emotions, whereas her mother continued her family's tradition of strict standards for behavior. Karen had never told them about her use of marijuana or the friends with whom she liked to 'party'. She never told them that she had received intermittent counseling for depression and had used antidepressant medication for two years until she discontinued about eight months ago.

When she felt upset or lonely, which happened daily, Karen tended to use alcohol. Alcohol had a 'warming and relaxing' effect and enabled her to behave more socially and with less anxiety than usual. She would often smoke marijuana by herself or with friends, saying this 'calms me down'. She wouldn't talk much to others when high on pot, but said she also did not care at those times. When she was not high, she would ruminate about how she did not feel at ease with others and her belief that others saw this and thought she was 'different'. She thought a great deal about being different, and these thoughts often included questions about her sexual orientation. She had been approached by women who wanted to date her, or who were friends but wanted to include a sexual experience in the friendship. Karen became involved for a time with one woman, but 'hadn't gone all that far' with her, and was not sure how far she wanted to move in this direction. She would date men on occasion, had sexual experiences with men, but had not felt deeply involved with any of these men. She felt attracted to men, but felt more relaxed and affectionate with women.

Karen's work in counseling revolved around the following focal areas: relationship with parents, clarification of sexual identity, coping with depression and anxiety, dealing with dependence on alcohol and marijuana, and finding new ways to address physical tension. These interrelated areas were addressed according to the way she formed figural gestalts, that is, according her expression of the development of meaning and her perceptions of significant events, emotions, or directions. The development of gestalts, or meaningful perceptual wholes, has been addressed by many theoreticians (e.g. Kohler 1929; Perls, Hefferline and Goodman 1951). Gestalt formation can be used to provide a conceptual bridge to Asian perspectives, particularly with the idea found in Taoism *that nature itself constructs meaningful wholes* by relating all apparently opposite conditions and qualities (Bryant 1993). A Taoist approach suggests that one allow one's true nature to follow its own course, without striving to make it fit predetermined categories or ways of being (Chan 1959; Rogers 1959; Watts 1960). This approach helped Karen accept her bisexual orientation and create meanings that 'fit' her experience and worldview.

The therapist assisted Karen's creative development of new meanings without providing predetermined resolutions or meanings. The Taoist perspective was incorporated into working with Karen by assuming that she would be better able to develop meaning if she were able to relax, and let go of strenuous efforts to 'make everything fit' or 'make everything make sense'. Therapy was useful to examine the predetermined meanings imposed by her family's culture and the larger culture, and to see how these predetermined meanings interfered with the meaning that was evolving 'of itself' from Karen's life experience. Allowing life and experience to 'be what it is', to unfold of itself without strain or self-conscious effort is a key in Taoist approaches (Moore 1983), and was a very useful attitude in therapy as Karen released herself from comparisons with others and grew in self-acceptance.

Karen was aware that she wanted change in dealing with negativity and anxiety. She discussed wanting to change her level of physical tension, and 'get past' the persistent doubts and negative thoughts about herself. However, she also feared change. In particular, she was concerned that if she changed this might require more honesty with her parents about her feelings, thoughts, and sexual orientation. She increasingly experienced herself as bisexual and this created a great deal of uncertainty for her. Karen suspected that her already strained relationship with parents might become extremely distant. One of her friends, who identified herself as a lesbian, had told Karen that Karen was 'for sure a lesbian' and she 'needed to come out' to really own this. Karen had thought about doing this, but was concerned about the effect this would have on friendships, work relationships, and her own sense of identity.

Her ability to verbalize her thoughts and feelings, to be aware of strengths, and to be open to possibilities for change were considered indicative that therapy would likely be fruitful. However, Karen noted that although she could notice and value positive aspects of self (e.g. 'it is important to me to be honest'), her mood and outlook might yet be maintained with negative feelings and extreme pessimism. For example, problems in family communications could become the basis for persistent anxiety and rumination around the theme of 'losing my family' to the point where sleep became difficult and the quality of her daily activities might be affected. She would struggle with persistent feelings of a self-negative and self-blaming nature in spite of thinking that these feelings weren't based on reality and ignored her strengths.

Conflict with her family intensified as Karen discussed some of her ideas about sexuality with them. Perhaps triggered by this family conflict, she expressed concern that symptoms of depression she experienced in the past had begun to recur. She was concerned with difficulties sleeping, lack of energy and motivation, appearing to others to be 'drifting off' during meetings at the administrative office where she held a part-time secretarial job. Although she experienced a shift toward greater self-acceptance and relaxation during the intitial phase of counseling, Karen decided to return to using a particular antidepressant medication which also lowered anxiety, and which she found had helped in the past. The question of medication was addressed as an option which she might choose or not, depending on her best decision after discussing potential benefits and costs. She perceived a cyclical, probably biological aspect to her cycles of mood, and saw medication as a means to regulate moods.

Having reached the decision to use an antidepressant, we framed this as a 'tool' to be used with the idea that she might reach a point where she was ready to move on without it. Although traditional Asian psychologies might have preferred herbal treatments for mood, Karen was a Western client living in the context of Western culture and its assumptions and 'tools'. The choice to use medication was congruent with her culture and we assumed that a holistic approach could include such a decision. We discussed, as a future option, decreasing and perhaps eliminating reliance on the medication if the 'timing were right'. This eventually came to pass, as Karen experienced increasing confidence in her own self-regulating abilities. She later began using a milder herbal supplement in place of the medication.

During the initial phase of counseling, Karen expressed a great deal of confusion regarding issues around sexual identity. She alternated between strong feelings of love and hate toward her parents. We worked together to allow her to accept these polarities of experience without feeling forced to choose a rigid stance toward her parents. Lack of clarity about her identity moved toward greater self-confidence and clarity of awareness as she was able to accept divergent feelings and perspectives that were included in her life experience.

At times in her counseling, Karen was assisted to develop her ability to relax by using full breathing, 'tuning in' to body awareness, and some use of imagery that assisted relaxation and self-acceptance. Substance use had allowed her to create temporary positive feelings that substituted for relaxation, self-acceptance, and positive feelings that might have come from being able to be honest with others and with oneself. Karen remarked about this, 'I feel like it's been such an effort to try to be honest with people who I don't see as being able to be honest with me. But at a certain point, I knew I had to be honest for me. It didn't change them, or the way they were dealing with things, but it changed me. And then it wasn't hard for me. When I knew I had to do it, then it became easy.' Additionally, Karen pursued two months of biofeedback work in addition to therapy (biofeedback was available to students in a lab associated with the counseling center). Biofeedback enabled Karen to receive moment-to-moment information about states of her body (e.g. skin temperature and electric discharge from muscles). This information was used to further Karen's ability to self-regulate physiological reactions.

Asian psychologies assume that reality can seem paradoxical when approached in words and concepts, and that conceptual polarities do not need to be seen as opposites (Chan 1963). With regard to Karen's treatment, polarities in emotions, and divergent ways of experiencing herself, were treated as acceptable and as facets of her identity. Rather than trying to force unification on her experience, Karen was allowed to discover unity for herself, through her ability to accept and use differing emotions and perspectives.

An assumption made in therapy was that Karen's holistic sense of congruence enhanced her well-being. That is, sensing an 'unsplit awareness' regulating congruent interaction between feelings, perceptions, actions, speech, and relationship was integral to health. This congruence could be addressed directly in counseling and supported as it occurred outside of counseling. As this integrated self-expression increased, Karen perceived that she was dealing with reality without having to distort or avoid. Clearly, this was an important function of counseling, because such ideas about facing reality were expressed by Karen regarding her feelings about sex and intimacy, about facing anxiety and feelings of weakness, and about what occurred in her family. Counseling assisted Karen to make her own determinations about what was best for her in an atmosphere that allowed her to safely consider options, express feelings, and acknowledge the validity of her perceptions.

Karen continued to practice breathing and relaxation 'on her own' while continuing to work on interpersonal and intrapsychic themes in counseling. Relaxation/meditation exercises were discussed as one way she could use focusing, relaxing, and 'letting go' as means to release herself from reliance on substances to control feelings. Other means Karen used included going for walks in the park, writing down thoughts as she sat by a lake near her house, and allowing herself to spend extra time enjoying taking a bath. She also learned to allow time for friends with whom she could 'just talk and be myself', and to regard this activity as an equally high priority as school work. Karen exercised when she was able, and reported positive effects when she was able to exercise three times a week. Periodically, her therapist 'checked in' with Karen regarding her balance of time between work and leisure activities, and the continuity of her relaxation practice.

THEMES FROM ASIAN PSYCHOLOGY

A perspective that integrates mind and body and treats the person holistically is an essential feature of Asian psychology. As we work in the West to develop a balanced approach that is grounded in Western cultural roots, we can find ways to integrate Asian ideas that can assist the development of a new vision of health and well-being. At the same time that some institutions have tended to supress such a change in orientation toward holism, a 'grassroots' movement has occurred that has supported the growth of a multibillion-dollar holistic health industry. Thus, millions of dollars are spent every month on alternative health-care practices and preventative measures such as meditation classes, massage therapy, acupuncture, herbs, and so on. Sometimes the offerings of this industry are questionable, yet the growth of the industry reflects a longing, associated with the desire for a holistic perspective; such longings and desires need to be addressed within traditional as well as non-traditional Western approaches. People in the West currently are expressing a longing for a non-dichotomizing approach to health and well-being (Weil 1988).

The model for Karen's treatment is developed from the Taoist understanding that polarized situations (for example, love versus hate, or individual versus family) involve one category (e.g. 'black') that defines another category (e.g. 'white'), while the first category is simultaneously being defined by the second (Watts 1966). This perspective invites us to take a wider view of reality. Thus, as a culture is defining an individual, the individual also defines the culture. As mental images affect bodily experience, bodily experience affects mental images. Aversion and desire arise together.

When therapy is conceptualized in terms of reciprocal definitions and interactions, we focus on understanding and working with mind and body as a process, rather than relying simply on isolated elements, such as chemicals, to define how moods are created. In working with this model, we find much support from worldviews presented in traditional Asian psychologies, particularly Buddhism and Taoism. Theorists such as Goleman (1976), Jung (1964), and Watts (1966) have recognized the following important postulate. The worldview presented in Asian psychology has more to do with understanding and promoting the resonance and harmony of interdependent factors than with using one factor to control and force change in other factors. Thus, the general worldview of Asian psychologies can be termed 'holistic' in the sense that the view of life and persons as whole, and as changing constantly within a context of wholeness and balance. This worldview is open to non-linear aspects of life and change, as well as more direct and linear connections, such as are the focus in most mainstream Western approaches to health and therapy.

Generally, the therapy process focuses on verbalization of experience and communication that demonstrates how one formulates interpretations and concepts from experience. Therapy can affect how experience is processed as well as how experience is interpreted and expressed. Asian psychology can contribute technical considerations that affect experiencing of self (e.g. the idea of observing one's breathing), and more importantly, can provide principles to guide therapeutic dialogue and the interaction of therapist with client. We now briefly consider how each of the ten principles we introduced earlier are therapeutically useful.

Compassion and empathy have been associated with growth in awareness and with therapeutic healing through relationship (Rogers 1980). Evident in therapy as an attitude that facilitates disclosure and intimacy, compassion may be viewed as a way to approach another and as a way of understanding. Rather than considering compassion a special condition involved between two beings (as perhaps 'romantic love' might be considered), Asian psychology suggests that the being of each living entity is considered as included in all, and all included in each (Watts 1972). To whatever extent this reality is sensed and is part of awareness, to that extent will a person naturally relate in a compassionate manner. Mutual awareness and respect that arises in the context of therapeutic relationship allows clients (and therapists as well) to enhance the ability for compassion toward self and others.

Compassion would best be considered not simply as something offered by the therapist toward the client but as a mutual recognition of a relationship that arises from the ground of awareness in which therapy is transacted. The therapist is assumed to have an awareness of how compassion can be expressed within relationship and how compassion might be considered as inherent to healing through a relationship. The therapist's awareness of this reality is an aspect of how therapy process develops, but it cannot develop unless and until the client engages and accepts the reality of compassion, particularly with regard to self, but also in consideration of self with others.

A central theme for Karen, as is the case for many clients in therapy, was her desire to give and receive love, compassion, and affection. Many clients will use therapy to assess ways that giving and receiving affection can work for them, apart from the definitions supplied by family or larger culture which have not worked. They may find new ways to invite affection and intimacy, and may or may not find methods to apply this to change family relationships. The therapeutic relationship can be considered a laboratory for the experiment of discovering new ways to express and receive contact between human beings. The Western spiritual concern with giving and receiving love in relationship with others can be considered a central principle that enters into healing and therapy (e.g. see Tillich 1980; Yalom 1980). If we understand the giving and receiving of love and empathy within a relationship as compatible with Eastern views about compassion and awareness, we find a key area for 'bridge-building' between Asian and Western psychology.

A compassionate and loving atmosphere provides acceptance and non-imposition of views of the other or the world. Non-imposition of views from the therapist allows a 'creative space' for a client to release old assumptions, change existing assumptions, or develop new views (Perls 1972; Rogers 1980). Valuing this creative space does not mean that views are not expressed or shared by the therapist. The interaction of therapy provides 'nutrients' that can be used by a client in gaining new self-definition, yet it is assumed that the client's work involves accepting what fits and rejecting what does not. Thus, the therapist may offer feedback or a perspective, but needs to check with the client whether this fits with the client's experience or is useful for the client. For example, a therapist might suggest that focus on breathing can assist self-regulation of stress and anxiety, a concept key in Asian psychology (Requena 1997). The therapist will then discover whether this approach is useful and how it is affecting a client. If the client does not find it useful, this assertion would be validated (rather than assume that in some way the client 'should' be able to benefit from this approach). Thus, self-definition through awareness is validated as a central principle, with respect for the client's ability to formulate self through experiential awareness.

Often, it will be discovered in therapy that the client is imposing views on herself. The work in therapy may be to determine from whence these 'internal voices' or 'messages' originated, and to assist the client to differentiate such messages from self. In other cases, no clear external source for negative self-messages is identified (e.g. culture or family), yet the client can be helped to see that when the self over-monitors the activities of self, confusion and negativity result. The therapist often models encouraging and supportive responses, thus suggesting that negative self-judgment, over-criticism and over-scrutiny of self are counterproductive. Confrontation can be an important aspect of therapy, but confrontation with feedback about aspects of functioning outside of usual awareness are most helpful when presented non-judgmentally and compassionately. The therapist suggests, 'you may look at this a new way' rather than 'you should be seeing this differently'.

It is assumed that the client can be (and must be) the judge of when and how to use information she or he received and shared in therapy. The client is the one in the situation, and in the best position to ascertain when and how to use learnings. This assumption is associated with an acknowledgment that the client is, or is learning, to be the authority on how to develop and support changes, and the one whose responsibility it is to decide if and when to implement such changes.

In Hindu and Buddhist thinking, the maintenance of patterns in thought and relationships is referred to as 'karma', and is considered an aspect of human individual and communal life. Karma is treated as the means to learn from experience, and as forming a web that connects individuals with communities through relationship patterns (Humphreys 1983). People grow as they become able to act in new ways that do not repeat negative past patterns of thinking and acting, as they find ways to heal hurts in relationships and generate compassion.

Balance of physiological aspects of lifestyle, such as sleeping, eating, exercise and leisure activities, can often affect mood issues that affect relationships. This holistic view of the person's health is consistent with the connection between mind, body, emotions and spirit postulated in Chinese and Japanese philosophy, exercise, and martial arts (Cheng 1981; Requena 1997; Stevens 1984). This concern for holistic well-being may be developed through experience of relaxation in one's life as well as 'inner' relaxation through self-acceptance and an open movement through experiencing of self and others. Education may be involved in discussing with clients how nutrition, sleep, exercise and leisure time affect the maintenance of resiliency, psychologically as well as physically.

The concept of balance becomes key when working with internal feeling states. Contradictory feelings and motivations are often presented as problems, and balance allows the person to encompass diverse feeling states without feeling 'torn'. Particularly difficult are contradictory experiences of self or significant others (e.g., valuing and devaluing). In the process of accepting these contradictory states, the person learns to trust his or her being. The individual learns experientially that 'things can turn out right' without making an effort to impose a solution, by accepting the process 'as is'. The relationship with substances, such as alcohol or marijuana, often simply mirrors the imbalanced feeling states experienced with significant others, such as family members. It is when the person finds balance within self that family relationships and relationships with substances can be redefined in ways that are healthy.

As an individual becomes aware of inherent wholeness, a natural release of self-negative thinking and feeling occurs. Thus, balancing leads to awareness of wholeness, and awareness of wholeness leads to a natural releasing process. The client is not exhorted to release negativity, this simply occurs naturally as wholeness is recognized. An individual who changes patterns of substance abuse is likely also to incur the loss of friends who 'hung out' with him to drink or get high. There may be the loss of a previous role one had with parents or peers, particularly if issues related to sexual orientation lead to a new sense of identity. These kinds of losses can be accepted constructively when such losses occur from a sense of oneself as intrinsically whole.

As clients perceive wholeness, they will naturally recognize those faulty assumptions about self that reflect unbalanced negativity, criticism, or perfectionistic expectations. Clients will sort out which ways of thinking and which roles will be maintained and which will be dropped. From an Eastern perspective, growing by releasing fixed concepts that anchor identity seems quite viable, whereas Western developmental theories seem to generally focus on developing a consistent and well-anchored identity as a prerequisite for mental health. Somewhat paradoxically (and as we saw with Karen), clients often become more consistent, clear, and coherent in their 'sense of self', as they become more comfortable in letting go of the previously perceived 'need' for a rigidly defined and predictable sense of self. This kind of growth seems to depend on finding a sense of 'inner stability' that does not depend on providing definitions of self to others. Asian psychologies, such as Buddhism and Taoism, indicate that our usual ideas of self are generally based on assumptions about constancy that are more imaginary than real.

Asian psychologies teach that attention, in and of itself, is valuable. Paying attention well is considered the basis for learning, growth, harmony, and changing one's consciousness from error to truth. This principle, applied to therapy, invites the therapist to construct a dialogue with the client that values awareness in and of itself. Through paying full attention to the nature of reality, one learns that ideas about reality depend on mood, situation, and role. Attention can help individuals to break with fixed ideas of how self or reality 'is supposed to be', thus taking persons 'out of themselves'. This giving of awareness over to experiencing allows new flexibility to emerge, yet with a new stability associated with clarity. Asian psychologies consider health and well-being to be associated with lack of self-consciousness or narcissistic self-involvements that interefere with the process of attending to events (Suzuki 1983).

The therapeutic process can be viewed as hinging on the collaborative abilities of client and counselor to attend to 'inner' and 'outer' events in counseling and in the client's life. Linking 'inner' with 'outer' was evident when Karen became able to link family relationships to inner feelings and expectations of herself. She could then form new links based on new ideas about herself, related to new ways of processing feelings and of relating to family members. All these developments were based on attention during therapeutic conversations, and outside of therapy. From this perspective, a client practices within therapy the kind of attention that will be valuable outside of therapy. This is attention to 'inner' feelings and perceptions and to 'outer' dialogue, communication, and exchange of energy.

Attention reveals that change already **is** occurring. Change does not need to be made to happen. Although clients (and all persons) inevitably deal with stress during times of accelerated change, clients can simultaneously develop new capacities for regulating stress. A key way to regulate the stress of change is to decrease resistance to change as an inherent aspect of reality. Acceptance of change as reality leads to appreciation of harmony within a situation of flux. Each person is a pattern of movement, not a fixed concrete entity. Acceptance of this fact is the beginning of appreciation for oneself and one's world as they are. In Taoism, such appreciation is linked to awareness that all things have their 'way', or their 'tao'. Thus, the 'Tao' of Karen, that is, the 'Way' of 'being Karen', became increasingly more effortless, spontaneous, and less restricted by self-consciousness and self-judgment (Bryant 1993). As she released the hold she had on trying to fit a certain image, she became more free to use her intuitions about what was right for her in specific situations and interactions, as well as in the overall picture of who she was in her lifespace. Her sense of wholeness increased as she became more flexible and did not need to fit into a mold defined by her family's or society's logic of what wholeness was supposed to be.

Asian psychologies indicate that health and well-being are associated with energy flowing in an unblocked manner (Requena 1997, Stevens 1984). Problems in living are linked to interference with the natural healthy flow of energy. Because mind and body are considered to be intimately connected, the flow of energy is assumed to affect mind and body. Proper attention facilitates energy flow, as does connection between mind and body, with an appropriately balanced lifestyle. When a client is able to attend in a balanced way to self, others, and environment, he or she might appropriately terminate therapy. Sometimes, as was the case with Karen, a client will leave therapy and return later to 'fine tune' the dynamically balanced attention they have developed. The work in therapy was to help her formulate a clear direction and movement for that theme, rather than to have it 'resolved' when she left counseling. If change is considered as ongoing, then the work of therapy is to have a client prepared to adapt, to be flexible, and to maintain balance when dealing with change, rather than having 'a completed change process' at the end of therapy.

Karen's work in therapy is typical of many clients, insofar as her work toward growth enabled her development of a more nondualistic framework to view herself and others. That is, change occurs as individuals no longer set a 'desirable' self against an 'undesirable' self, or 'good' attitudes and feelings against 'bad' attitudes or feelings. Growth through acceptance of contradictory feelings, experiences, and perspectives could be said to lead to appreciation of paradox in life while experiencing self more simply, nondefensively, and openly. From a Western psychological perspective, we might say the client becomes more 'integrated'. From an Asian perspective, we might say clients have released some of the self-imposed blocks to knowing self as 'originally whole' (Watts 1975). Self-acceptance enables individuals to tolerate and, at times, to enjoy the differing feelings, reactions, and perspectives that can be included as 'self'.

ASIAN PSYCHOLOGY'S CONTRIBUTION TO WESTERN APPROACHES TO HEALTH PSYCHOLOGY

Viewing health as a holistic process that depends on the movement of energy might be construed as a central contribution of Asian psychology. Finding out where the flow of energy is 'blocked' would then be a greater key to assisting clients than finding the correct DSM IV diagnosis. Four patterns that might indicate blocked energy would include: (1) intellectualization (when energy is focused too intently on ideas and concepts to the detriment of other necessary uses and expressions of energy, such as processing emotion or sensation and/or using physical movement), (2) compulsive or addicted patterns of energy expression (blocking open awareness and spontaneous reactions to situations as they arise), (3) fear of asserting ideas, emotions, or perceptions (when energy is inhibited from involvement in development and expression of thoughts and perceptions), and (4) noncontactful relationship processes (either inhibited, disengaged or intrusive use of self in relationship; pulling back or overextending one's energy such that fluid and 'contactful' relational processes are not formed).

Asian psychologies tend to assume that if harmony of energy flow can be established, health and well-being will follow (Requena 1997). Thus, in Chinese T'ai Ch'i exercises, the flow of ch'i or organic energy is emphasized (Cheng 1981). Hindu theories of health refer to this flow as the movement of 'prana' through breathing or 'kundalini' as it moves up the spine to the brain (Krishna 1997). Japanese systems of martial arts, influenced by Chinese ideas about 'chi',refer to 'ki' energy (Stevens 1984). In Western psychology, we may develop a more holistic view of the health of persons as we increasingly recognize that the person has natural and inherent resources to move toward balance if he or she can be assisted to release self-imposed blockage to the movement of energy.

In the West, concern with the movement of energy can be traced back to Freud, who saw repression as a blockage of natural energy that yearned to connect with 'objects' (i.e. people) in the environment. Freud's view of libido has similarities with concepts such as 'chi' or 'kundalini', which are discussed in terms of transmutation of sexual energy, much as Freud saw sublimation (Brill 1976). Whereas Freud stressed the importance of controlling and consciously directing this energy, Carl Rogers (1980) stressed that we need to learn to trust this energy and its natural directions. He asserted that if the right conditions were provided in therapy, the client would naturally self-direct toward growth in whatever ways were most effective for that client. Asian writings seem to have an ability to reconcile these apparently opposite kinds of awareness (i.e. that our intrinsic energy needs to be controlled and directed, and that it can be trusted). In general, Asian teachers of meditation, healing, or martial arts tend toward a more 'directive' stance than Rogers as they facilitate their students' growth in awareness (e.g. through meditation or exercises), yet Asian teachers also seem to be more trusting of 'unconscious' wisdom than Freud.

Asian psychologies tend to include an educative and somewhat authoritative role for the teacher, who is assumed to be able to sense where energy might be blocked, and to have knowledge of how to release these blocks. Asian teachers may assume that their way of interacting will turn out 'right' because their attunement to energy is 'right'. One conclusion from looking at these issues is that no predetermined formula of being directive or nondirective will suffice to address ways to unblock energy for individual clients. Another conclusion is that the therapist's work on self will be a key ingredient, as energy that is blocked for the therapist will affect the process of therapy in ways that may inhibit the client's ability to unblock energy and release limiting assumptions.

Asian psychologies' trust of the natural movement of energy has relevance to Freud's ideas about therapy, as opposed to his ideas about psychopathology. Freud believed that therapy should be practiced by decreasing self-censorship, allowing associations to occur freely, and decreasing the overly punitive messages of the 'superego' or internalized and rigid social conscience (Brill 1976). All these techniques encouraged internal energy to move more freely. One difference between Freud's theory and Asian approaches is that Asian theories tend to view the unconscious as the seat of spiritual growth as well as the basis for desires and biological energies (Suzuki 1983). This assumption in Asian psychologies implies that learning to 'let oneself be' is a life-affirming approach rather than a passive or self-indulgent approach (which might be the conclusion from some Western perspectives). Associated with this Asian idea is the recognition (a key aspect of Taoist thought) that non-imposition of conceptual judgments and expectations is a necessary perquisite for truly life-affirming awareness (Bryant 1993; Chan 1963). Growth occurs when the timing is right, not by forcing or demanding growth nor by trying to make some ideal condition come to be.

Therapy can be seen as similar to the 'pushing hands' exercise in T'ai Ch'i 's view of energy as applied to martial arts. Pushing hands involves sensing the energy of the opponent, yielding when the opponent extends, pushing where the opponent is unstable, maintaining one's own balance, remaining grounded, remaining close enough to sense energy yet with enough distance not to be 'taken over' by the other (Cheng 1981). The therapist who applies these principles will value the sensing of energy that occurs in personal encounters. The therapist will allow himself or herself to be affected by the client's energy, but not in ways that would destabilize or unground the therapist. Contact will be maintained, allowing the client to express what is emerging, yet not simply allowing this expression to occur in a void. The therapist remains present, in touch with what is expressed, responding in ways that maintain contact and allow the therapist, when appropriate, to move forward into areas which may usually be avoided or ignored (the 'unstable' areas of the client's structure of awareness). This movement can be done in a way that maintains integrity and respect while, when appropriate, challenging limitations or rigidities in the client's system of dealing with internal energy. Because energy dynamics are involved in the therapeutic relationship, changing how energy is exchanged in the context of the therapeutic dialogue can lead to changes in relationships outside of therapy.

A key concept in Buddhism is that reality is a constant changing of conditions, thus leading to the conclusion that not being attached to any particular condition is the basis for psychological freedom (Humphreys 1983). Balance must be attained within the process of change rather than be imposed upon change. This contribution leads to different assumptions than those employed by most Western approaches. Western models tend to generate a predetermined 'way to do things' that leads to certain predictable and expected outcomes. Although Asian models can be viewed as postulating desired outcomes (e.g. enlightenment), they emphasize a process in which awareness is key and in which order is generated from awareness as it is in the process of change. Thus, although enlightenment is desirable, it is an already present reality, not something to strive for (Suzuki 1983; Watts 1966). With regards to therapeutic work, Asian models suggest that we should be open to working with what is emerging within consciousness as it is apprehended and experienced by clients. The appropriate movement of energy is valued whereas the client's ability to introject and impose the proper concepts upon experience is not valued.

Because energy is assumed to be an essentially unitive phenomenon, working with clients involves not 'taking sides' when dealing with clients' internal oppositions. For example, rather than imposing a conceptual scheme designed to minimize anxiety, Asian meditative traditions suggest 'being with the anxiety', observing it, allowing it to be there until it changes. Change is assumed to come 'of itself', as part of the way reality works. Perls (1972) was influenced by such Asian concepts, and tried to formulate a therapy in which he would expose both sides of a polarity without aligning with either side. Thus, taking sides against one aspect of an internal opposition cannot lead to holistic balance and might even create additional blockage or fragmentation of the movement of energy. This approach implies that a therapist will do better work if her or she is not conceiving of clients in split ways (e.g. not trying to avoid some aspects of a client's experience, nor distorting perceptions of a client's experiences to fit the therapist's preconceived categories).

A final contribution of Asian thought that is important to mention is the view that a self-centered approach to reality inevitably leads to distortion, ignorance, and conflict (Chan 1963). The Asian approach generally does not to try to impose a non-self-centered way of doing things. Rather, people are encouraged to gain new awareness that changes the limiting and constricting worldview centered around the separate self (Watts 1966). Ultimately, the separate self is no longer there as the basis for awareness. This approach differs from Western thought concerning the extent of the change that it views as possible for human awareness. The concerns of Western psychology are generally more 'worldly', more concerned with living an effective life, grounded in the abilities to work and love (as Freud postulated). An integration of European–American and Asian psychologies would likely lead to an approach that addressed the concerns of living effectively in the world while 'knowing oneself', yet understanding that growth also involves an 'unknowing of self' that can leads to total change of one's worldview. Most clients in therapy enter counseling because of worldly concerns. Through addressing these concerns, they can be assisted to know themselves with more clarity, and 'unknow' themselves in the sense of letting go obsolete assumptions and expectations.

An integration of Western and Eastern concerns lead to a view that knowing oneself and 'unknowing' oneself are twin aspects of one movement of being/becoming. The best way to be able to evolve within this movement depends, to a great extent, on what is right for a person as an individual, based on his or her particular context, history, and energy. In working with clients, it is possible to meet the client where he or she is, that is, to base the therapeutic approach on the client's worldview and subjective experience of needs and wants. If this is done, the therapy will not impose either a 'worldly' or 'spiritual' goal on a client with disregard to what fits the client's own experience and perception.

Asian concepts of change can help Western thought become more flexible when addressing the Western value of developing a strong, consistent, and more adaptable self. Change can be viewed as depending on a letting go of the previous self as much as depending on a formulation of new constructs. If 'letting go' is emphasized, then therapy will tend to include open-ended inquiry as a process rather than focusing on constructing linear paths to goals. This kind of integration is possible, but challenging, in the current climate in Western health-care delivery (which in many settings requires clearly delineated observable goals in order to receive reimbursement). We may address goals for practical reasons, yet value qualities such as openness, awareness of feelings and intuitions, and awareness of the unknown within our experience. The value we place on these latter qualities is in the service of creating a healing dialogue, which is less likely to occur in the absence of these qualities and with only a linear focus on goal attainment.

Although reimbursement of therapy may depend largely on goal achievement, therapy as healing the whole person depends more on enlarging and focusing awareness than on creating a dialogue that is a means to an end. Acknowledging and observing 'inner' and 'outer' events is more essential than 'fixing' or 'removing' problems, although wanting to solve a problem often is the focus that brings a client to therapy. Problems can be solved in the process of expanding awareness, rather than by applying mechanical formulae. Such solutions, because they are generated from growing awareness, are likely to be more appropriate, and lead to confidence that one can generate one's own solutions.

EASTERN AND WESTERN VIEWS OF THE SELF

A major implication about the nature of the self that differentiates Eastern and Western thought is this: Western thought strongly validates the idea that the self is a stable entity that exists and develops over time, and around which meaning is organized. Eastern thought validates the idea that the self arises in a relational manner within the present moment of experience and does not have any ultimately separable existence. Western personality theory, developmental theories, and psychotherapies focus on how we develop successful and healthy selves versus neurotic and dysfunctional selves. Eastern theories focus on how to constructively 'lose the self'. No integration between Western and Eastern ideas will truly work unless these concerns can be brought into relationship with each other in a unified manner. To the extent that Western psychology and therapy has viewed the self as a bounded cognitive and perceptual entity that is imposed on experience, the Western view is not compatible with the Eastern view. This integration would then call for a revision of Western therapy and theory toward a more relational and creative view of the self. Issues such as human development, the nature of human personality, and definitions of health and well-being are likely to be affected. Related questions will need to be addressed about the pursuits around which Western culture is currently oriented (e.g. pursuit of personal profit, aggrandizement, status and consumption as fundamental to social structure).

Hopefully, the integration we are proposing can lead to a view of the healthy self as grounded in non-self-centered compassionate awareness. Compassion is an attitude toward contact with other living beings that is closely aligned with the idea of empathy. Empathy can be found as an essential element of Person-Centered therapy (Rogers 1980) and Self Psychology (Kohut 1977), and many other existential and psychoanalystic writings. Thus, we have seen evidence of this concern emerging in Western thought for some time.

Asian approaches teach us that meaning arises from an aspect of the self that we cannot accurately put into words, and therefore to which we cannot assign conceptual meaning. Unlike Freud's ideas about the unconscious,

Asian approaches regard the non-conceptualized aspect of self as intelligent, aware, and fundamentally creative. The Western therapeutic construct that seems closest to this ability of the self to construe verbal meanings from a nonverbal source of awareness might be 'intuition'. In application to therapy, we gain new freedom to utilize the concepts of timing, silent aware-ness, and using intuition to form meanings and directions. Spontaneously 'knowing what to do' without having to think about it can be encouraged as a valuable part of therapy.

A person being asked to reflect about what she said or did in a session might be able to explain part of the process. But at the time, she did or said what 'came naturally'. This intuitive process of reacting to present events seems more validated in Asian psychologies such as Zen Buddhism or Tao-ism than in Western approaches that require logical explanation as the basis for taking an action. From a Taoist perspective, for example, overreliance on logic and words to formulate actions is a kind of split-mindedness that causes an artificial gap to arise between the person and present experience, the individual and the Tao of life. Mastery of the Tao is considered evident when a person can act without depending on selfconscious reflection. Spon-taneous actions, based on intuition, then occur in ways that fit the situation perfectly, without hesitation or error.

One cannot act with one's awareness 'in the moment' if one is fighting against spontaneity. The psychologies of Taoism and Buddhism advocate a total acceptance of the present moment, awareness of 'what is' without separation of subject from object, or awareness from reality. This nonsepara-tion is not a 'primitive fusion' in which the self cannot act, but rather a 'unified field' in which sophisticated action and awareness is possible (Wil-ber 1980). In application to therapy, this principle was used with Karen to assist her to validate her full awareness of herself, her experience, her reac-tions, her wants, and her wishes.

For most clients, gaining a more holistic sense of self as they move through life, beginning to validate their intrinsic wholeness, is an adequate goal for therapy. At more advanced levels of study of the Tao, or of Buddha consciousness, goals are released. The person then finds beauty and reality in the moment to moment experience of 'what is', without any need to change things or fix things. Indeed, the intention to change to achieve a goal would be seen at this 'higher' level of awareness as the perpetuation of a split in awareness. Although clients in therapy usually would not be work-ing directly toward a realization of the Tao, they indirectly move toward it as they more fully accept who they are, and as they realize greater satisfac-tion and effectiveness through such acceptance. Because Western culture tends to indoctrinate its members in a splitting of thought from feeling, many clients come to therapy suffering from feelings they cannot control, or which will not submit to their concepts of how they 'should' feel. An Asian perspective validates working in therapy by not opposing feelings, rather by 'being with' them. The 'solution' provided in therapy then would not be newer and better ways to control feelings, but a greater and more unified awareness of self that includes feelings in a balanced way.

CONCLUSION

The model of counseling and well-being presented in this chapter is based on the concept of intrinsic wholeness. It is assumed that a person who is aware of reality will recognize self as non-separate from life. The person might then express a natural compassion based on sharing the source of being, the Tao, with others and with nature. From this perspective, compassion cannot be viewed merely as an 'element' of human functioning or even one of the 'core conditions' for effective therapy or living, but rather as a basic and pervasive aspect of the realization of reality. If awareness **is** reality in Asian psychology, and awareness without compassion is seen as unreal, then compassion must be necessary to reality. Without compassion, awareness moves away from itself and becomes ignorance.

In the Asian psychologies that we have discussed, compassion is simply present when reality is apprehended without the blinders of ignorance. In application to therapy, the therapist is compassionate, to whatever degree this occurs, because the interconnection of the client and therapist is evident. That is, compassion is not a quality that is modeled or provided by the therapist to facilitate good therapy or to reach certain goals (although compassion does facilitate and does move toward relatedness). Compassion is essential to the functioning of awareness in relationship, and is basic to the client and counselor being able to 'see' themselves and each other in the relationship as they are. Good therapy does tend to awaken compassion toward self and others through the quality of awareness involved in the dialogue. The therapeutic use of self is therefore the essential basis for good therapy in the integrative model which we are examining. Therapeutic use of self is not a technique, but a prerequisite for a relationship that allows awareness to heal. Healing occurs through relatedness and interaction, not through imposition of a model of health on the persons involved. The healing involved in psychotherapy occurs as compassion is awakened, in the client, in the therapist, and between the client and therapist.

We have shown ten principles derived from the view that awareness as such is the basis for movement toward health and well-being. Health and well-being arise from awareness, as the wholeness of awareness is expressed in compassionate relationship, balanced lifestyles, and sense of self as intrinsically whole. The intrinsic wholeness of self necessitates that 'the other' is included in self. The 'other' that is not separate from self may be construed as the body, the other person, the community, the group of outsiders, or nature. Thus, provision of health services requires awareness. Providing healing modalities as technologies is an insufficient approach. Technologies can be provided while the underlying awareness is not addressed. What is called for is service delivery that grows from a vision of well-being that includes other with self. Ultimately, the healing of society is implied in the healing of individuals. The reunification of the human community is necessitated by the inference that compassionate relationship is the basis for holistic healing.

REFERENCES

Brill, A.A. (1976) *Basic Principles of Psychoanalysis*. Westport, CT: Greenwood Press.

Bryant, B. (1993) In and out the Gestalt pail. *Gestalt Journal*, 16, 45–86.

Chan, W. (Ed. & Trans.) (1963) *A Source Book in Chinese Philosophy*. Princeton, NJ: Princeton University Press.

Cheng, M. (1981) *T'ai chi ch'uan*. Berkeley, CA: North Atlantic Books.

Dalai Lama (Bstan-dzin-rgya-mtsho, Dalai Lama XIV) (1997) *The Buddha Nature: Death and eternal soul in Buddhism*. Woodside, CA: Bluestar Communications.

Epstein, M. (1995) *Thoughts without a Thinker*. New York: Basic Books.

Ferlinghetti, L. (1958) *A Coney Island of the Mind: Poems*. New York: New Directions.

Ginsberg, A. (1959) *Howl, and other Poems*. San Francisco, CA: City Lights Books.

Goleman, D. (1976) Meditation and consciousness.: An Asian approach to mental health. *American Journal of Psychotherapy*, 30, 41–54.

Goleman, D. (1981) Buddhist and Western psychology: Some commonalities and differences. *Journal of Transpersonal Psychology*, 13, 125–136.

Goleman, D. and Schwartz, G.E. (1976) Meditation as an intervention in stress reactivity. *Journal of Consulting and Clinical Psychology*, 44, 456–466.

Humphreys, C. (1983) *Karma and Rebirth*. Wheaton, IL: Theosophical Publishing House.

Jung, C.G. (1964) *Man and his Symbols*. Garden City, NY: Doubleday.

Kerouac, J. (1958) *The Dharma Bums*. Cutchogue, NY: Buccaneer Books.

Kohler, W. (1929) *Gestalt Psychology*. New York: H. Liveright.

Kohut, H. (1977) *The Restoration of the Self*. New York: International Universities Press.

Krishna, G. (1997) *Kundalini*. Boston, MA: Shambhala.

Maslow, A.H. (1971) *The Farther Reaches of Human Nature*. New York: Viking Press.

Moore, N. (1983) The archetype of the Way: I. Tao and individuation. *Journal of Analytical Psychology*, 28, 119–140.

Murphy, G. and Murphy, L. (Eds) (1968) *Asian Psychology*. New York: Basic Books.

Perls, F. (1972) *In and Out the Garbage Pail*. New York: Bantam Books.

Perls, F. S., Hefferline, R.F. and Goodman, P. (1951) *Gestalt Therapy; Excitement and growth in the human personality*. New York: Julian Press.

Requena, Y. (1997) *Chi Kung*. Rochester, VT: Healing Arts Press.

Reynolds, D.K. (1984) *Playing Ball on Running Water: Living Morita psychotherapy: the Japanese way to build a better life*. New York: William Morrow.

Rogers, C. (1980) *A Way of Being*. Boston, MA: Houghton Mifflin.

Stevens, J. (1984) *Aikido, the Way of Harmony*. Boston, MA: Shambhala.

Suzuki, D.T. (1983) *An Introduction to Zen Buddhism*. London: Rider.

Tillich, P. (1980) *The Courage to Be*. New Haven, CT: Yale University Press.

Watts. A. (1966) *The Book, on the Taboo against knowing who you are*. New York: Vintage.

Watts, A. (1972) *The Supreme Identity; an essay on Oriental metaphysic and the Christian religion*. New York: Pantheon Books.

Watts, A. (1975) *Psychotherapy, East and West*. New York: Vintage Books.

Weil, A. (1997) *Eight Weeks to Optimum Health*. New York: A.A. Knopf.

Weil, A. (1988) *Health and Healing*. Boston, MA: Houghton Mifflin.

Welwood, J. (1996) Reflection and presence: The dialectic of self-knowledge. *Journal of Transpersonal Psychology*, 28, 107–128.

Wilber, K. (1980) *The Atman Project: A transpersonal view of human development*. Wheaton, IL: Theosophical Publishing House.

Yalom, I. (1980) *Existential Psychotherapy*. New York: Basic Books.

Chapter 7

Cultivating Health Through Complementary Medicine

Adrian Furnham and Charles Vincent

Complementary medicine is now widely used in Europe, North America and Australasia. In 1983 Fulder estimated that in Britain one medical consultation in ten was with a complementary practitioner of some kind (Fulder and Munro 1985). Since then interest in complementary medicine has grown and the number of complementary patients and practitioners has dramatically increased, though exact figures are diffcult to obtain. In the United States an estimated one in three people used an unconventional therapy in 1991, and the number of visits made to unconventional therapists exceeded those to all US primary care physicians (Eisenberg, Kessler and Foster 1993).

The fact that so many people currently choose to attend complementary practitioners suggests that they are receiving something that is important to them. Some complementary techniques may, as we will discuss, be of direct therapeutic benefit. However, whatever the benefits of the specific therapies, the phenomenon of complementary medicine has a great deal to teach us about the ingredients of a successful therapeutic relationship and the factors that assist or delay recovery from illness.

To illustrate some of the main themes of the chapter, and of research into complementary medicine, we present two case studies. Both are true accounts, the first extracted from a newspaper story and the second a slightly modified version of an account given to one of the authors.

Cultivating Health: Cultural Perspectives on Promoting Health. Edited by M. MacLachlan.
© 2001 John Wiley & Sons Ltd.

CASE STUDIES

PAULINE'S STORY

'I was seventeen when I first experienced the misery embodied in the word "cystitis": the dreadful urge to pee every five minutes and the ghastly pain and burning. I was rapped over the knuckles by my GP for being promiscuous and packed off to the local VD clinic—despite being a virgin. So began an intimate relationship with my urinary tract that was to last a quarter of a century. Self-help routines such as peeing after sex and drinking gallons of water laced with bicarb limited the attacks to between four and six a year. But when push came to shove, antibiotics were the only answer.

Last winter I went down with pneumonia. Seven weeks and three courses of antibiotics later, I was just beginning to stagger up and down stairs when there it was, the unmistakable dragging pain; the cystitis bacteria were back in business. I struggled on with the usual over-the-counter remedies—most of them variations on "pot.cit." [potassium citrate]—but it was no good, my resistance was too low. Ten days later my GP reluctantly prescribed the old standby, more antibiotics. But no sooner came relief than a relapse. This time no effect at all.

As well as the physical symptoms the sense of unease that always accompanied my attacks was by now verging on paranoia. I found myself seriously depressed and weeping hysterically over a boyfriend's illusory love affair; clearly I was in a bad way. A hospital appointment was made. The consultant was as sympathetic as anyone can be who has never been there. His diagnosis, if lacking in tact, was graphic: camel bladder, he called it. Over the years mine had stretched, and like an old balloon had lost its elasticity. As a result it never completely emptied but left that little soupçon behind, bursting with bacteria, all ready to infect the next intake of pee. He could offer no cure, but a prophylactic dose of antibiotics would keep the bacteria at bay, he said. Four times a day. For ever. Desperation overrode scepticism and I did as I was told. Then, two months later, a different set of symptoms broke cover. Same nether region, but this time the raw, dry itching of thrush. Thanks to the effectiveness of the antibiotics, candida yeasts were now up and at it and driving me mad. I stopped the pills. Within hours the cystitis was back.

A friend who believes antibiotics should carry a health warning persuaded me to try homeopathy. The first consultation cost £50, subsequent visits £25. Each time produced lots of chat, a new remedy, but no change.

By now I was completely incapacitated. My hot water bottle came with me everywhere. I even drove the car with it stuffed down my trousers. The thrush was back and, just to put the boot in, I had piles now, too. A full house. What about acupuncture, another friend asked. He could put me in touch with someone really good. Well, why not? I was at the end of the road.

Janine spent an hour going through my medical history. She took my pulses (each organ has its own, apparently) and found that the lower part of my body was colder than the rest. Had I noticed? Well, yes. The hot water bottle. It's what acupuncturists call damp heat, she told me, a significant cause being antibiotics. The cystitis, thrush, even the piles—everything was connected. All that was needed was a simple adjustment of my thermostat.

I don't know where she put the needles, I didn't watch. Somewhere on my left arm, I think. But, bizarre and irrational though it all was, I left feeling calm and well. That was in early November. Since then I have not had the slightest ache, twinge, sting or itch. It has gone. Just like that.

I have suffered too long to advise anyone to throw caution (i.e. pot.cit., yogurt or bicarb) to the wind. But if any of this nightmare rings bells, then it might be worth putting conventional medicine on hold. It is important not to forget that this is just **my** story and **my** happy ending. All I can say for sure is that for me it was without a doubt the best £35 I have ever spent, even though my fingers are still firmly crossed.'

PETER'S STORY

Peter was a 45-year-old divorcee living in Paris. He was a talented biologist and was interested in unorthodox scientific ideas about animal communication and ecological progress. He was lean, handsome and fit, when he collapsed suddenly at work. When he awoke three days later, he was very quickly told he had cancer of the brain. Orthodox cancer treatment began almost immediately with chemotherapy. An introvert, diffident but clever man, Peter began to research his condition. Reluctantly he continued with therapy prescribed by the Parisian doctors. But surfing the net, Peter found information about an unorthodox cure offered by a Canadian doctor which seemed to offer a reasonable chance of success. Despite the fact that he was not at all well, off Peter flew to Canada, took the complementary medical treatment and met other sufferers with his condition. He was impressed by what he saw, felt better and even went so far as to try to start a self-help group for patients with the same cancer.

The complementary therapy was 'holistic'. It involved changes in diet, lifestyle and how one perceived the world. Peter found it attractive because it fitted so well his own view of things. He was widely read, with degrees in biology, philosophy and psychology, and found that he could integrate ideas from many different fields—physics, medicine, psychology etc.

Peter continued both orthodox and complementary medicine at the same time, but he came to dislike the orthodox treatment more and more. He lost his hair, felt constantly tired and found the side effects of chemotherapy debilitating and unpleasant—'like having a bad hangover with a heavy cold'. He also felt that some of the doctors and nurses were arrogant or patronising, dismissive of his interest in complementary medicine. He was shocked by apparently how lacking in inquisitiveness they were, accepting the canons of orthodox medicine so unquestioningly, despite the fact that so many forms of cancer seemed 'incurable'. On the other hand, he felt patronised by some medics who treated his questions about the mechanisms and processes of the cure with disdain.

Some of the nurses he encountered were very kind, but he began to feel they all thought he was soon to die.

The experience of the complementary treatment could not have been a more dramatic contrast. Rather than feeling sick and depressed, he felt elated after the sessions. He was not uncritical or desperate, though, and thought that some of the 'mixtures' he had to take both unpleasant and unproven as to their efficacy. But he felt calmer after the consultation and felt that there was something he could to do help himself. He felt more in control of his destiny and also thought he felt well.

Peter e-mailed many other sufferers and became knowledgeable about not only brain cancer but also orthodox cures. He felt they were too insensitive, too gross: that there must be better ways than surgery or massive doses of chemicals to kill the cancerous cells. His relapse was sudden. Three weeks after he started feeling distinctly unwell he died. Two weeks before his death, he agreed to have brain surgery as a last hope. He knew that it was bound to leave long-lasting damage. He lost his ability to speak and his last days were doubly unhappy as he could not even communicate his anger and pain.

At a memorial service, people noted how much he felt the doctors had let him down. One person pointed to the thick files of cuttings and data they found at his home about brain cancer and all forms of cancer treatment. One of the mourners was herself a victim of the disease and one of the people Peter had networked with on the web. She spoke eloquently about Peter and the benefits derived from the complementary therapy in which he put so much faith. She said that though complementary therapy—and orthodox treatment—had clearly failed to halt the disease, it had obviously helped him. He felt calmer and optimistic after each treatment session.

As Pauline Dening says, this is just her story and her happy ending. One cannot draw any definite conclusions about the general efficacy of either orthodox or complementary treatment from either case. However, these accounts contain a number of important themes.

First, the content and tone of these accounts challenge various obstinate stereotypes that are sometimes invoked of the patient who seeks complementary treatment. Neither person appears to be stupid, naive, credulous or dismissive of orthodox medicine. Nor do they appear to be neurotic by nature, though illness brought misery and depression in both cases.

Second, both people failed to obtain relief of symptoms by conventional means, and this was a primary reason for turning to complementary medicine.

Third, the accounts are a warning not to equate all forms of complementary medicine, in terms of underlying philosophy, methods, or the behaviour of practitioners. For instance homeopathy was ineffective in Pauline's case, while acupuncture, scepticism notwithstanding, appears to have been effective. One or two sessions of acupuncture proved successful after years of antibiotics and a course of homeopathic treatment. The natural progress of disease, 'tincture of time', is sometimes invoked as the explanation of the apparent success of complementary treatments. Here this seems improbable; the improvement is too rapid, and the history too long. Acupuncture was effective or, at least some other concurrent factor or advice from the acupuncturist might have been responsible; reducing antibiotics, taking more rest or whatever.

Fourth, we can consider what other aspects of the therapeutic encounter might have provided a stimulus towards change. Peter found some of the doctors and nurses arrogant and patronising, in contrast to the sympathetic and open-minded approach of complementary practitioners he consulted. In Ms Dening's case the initial session with the acupuncturist was long, the history appears to have been detailed, and there was a careful physical examination. The acupuncturist was sympathetic and attentive. Yet the consultant is also described as 'as sympathetic as anyone can be'.

Fifth, there is the actual system of medicine and the explanation it provides for the patient. The acupuncturist asks Pauline whether she has noticed that part of her body is cold, and links various previously largely unconnected symptoms to a single basic imbalance. Understanding a variety of symptoms in terms of a single concept is, of course, equally a part of orthodox medicine; the suggestion is simply that it is important, not unique to complementary medicine.

Finally, for both Peter and Pauline, the sessions left them feeling 'calm and well'. The immediate experience of the treatment was positive, providing hope for the future and perhaps also indicative of enduring change.

COMPLEMENTARY MEDICINE AND COMPLEMENTARY THERAPIES

The term complementary medicine embraces a wide range of diverse therapies and diagnostic methods. Previous terms have included fringe medicine, unconventional medicine, unorthodox medicine, natural medicine and, the most widely used, alternative medicine. Complementary medicine is now the preferred description as practitioners of these therapies now see them as supplementing rather than replacing orthodox medicine.

A British Medical Association report (1986) listed 116 different types of complementary therapy and diagnostic aid. It is possible to classify the specialities along a number of dimensions: their history; the extent to which they have been professionalized; whether or not they involve touch; the range and type of disorders/problems they supposedly cure. The list of recognized CM therapies grows continually, but the list shown in Table 7.1 is reasonably comprehensive.

The history, philosophy and methods of treatment of even the main forms of complementary therapy are extremely diverse. The origins of some, for example acupuncture, are ancient while osteopathy and homeopathy date from the nineteenth century. Some (acupuncture, homeopathy) are complete systems of medicine, while others are restricted to diagnosis alone (iridology), or to a specific therapeutic technique (massage). The range of

Table 7.1 Complementary therapies

Acupuncture	Colour therapy	Osteopathy
Acupressure	Crystal and gem therapy	Ozone therapy
Alexander Technique	Dance movement therapy	Reiki
Aromatherapy Art therapy	Healing Herbal medicine	Reflexology Relaxation
Autogenic training	Homoeopathy	Shiatsu
Ayurveda	Hypnosis	Spiritual healing
Bach flower remedies	Magnetic therapy	Talk therapies, counselling
Biochemical tissue salts	Massage	Traditional Chinese medicine
Biorhythms	Meditation	Therapeutic touch
Chiropractic	Music therapy	Visualization
Chelation and cell therapy	Naturopathy	Voice and sound therapy
Colonic irrigation	Nutritional therapy	Yoga

treatments is equally varied: diet, plant remedies, needles, minuscule homeopathic doses, mineral and vitamin supplements and a variety of psychological techniques. The theoretical frameworks and underlying philosophy vary in coherence, complexity, and the degree to which they could be incorporated into current scientific medicine. Complementary practitioners vary enormously in their attitude to orthodox medicine, the extent of their training and their desire for professional recognition. There are, however, within this diversity, some broad common themes: a vitalistic philosophy embracing the idea of an underlying energy or vital force; a belief that the body is self-healing, and so a respect for minimal interventions; general, all-encompassing theories of disease and a strong emphasis on the prevention of disease and the attainment of positive health. While in much conventional medicine the patient is the passive recipient of external solutions, in complementary medicine the patient is more likely to be an active participant in regaining health (Vincent and Furnham 1997).

THE USE OF COMPLEMENTARY MEDICINE

The principal reasons for beginning CM are that it is more natural, effective and allows a more active role for the patient and second, the failure of orthodox medicine to provide relief for that specific complaint. The adverse effects of orthodox medicine, and a more positive patient–practitioner relationship are also important for many patients (Vincent and Furnham 1996). Patients of CM tend to be female, well educated and of higher than average social class. There is little to support the widely held view that complementary patients are especially gullible or naive, or have unusual (neurotic) personalities or (bizarre) value systems. However, comparisons of users and non-users of CM have shown evidence of different beliefs about health and disease. There is some evidence that they are more health conscious and believe more strongly that people can influence their own state of health, both by life-style and through maintaining a psychological equilibrium. Complementary patients appear to have less faith in 'provider control', that is, in the ability of medicine to resolve problems of ill health (Vincent, Furnham and Willsmore 1995; Vincent and Furnham 1997). Some studies of cancer patients using CM have found that they were more likely to believe cancer was preventable through diet, stress reduction and environmental changes and to believe that patients should take an active role in their own health (Downer *et al.* 1994). However, the results are quite clear: the increasing number of CM patients are not particularly unrepresentative of the population as a whole.

Complementary therapies are extremely widely used, and there is increasing interest and increasing demand. In the United States Eisenberg, Kessler and Foster (1993) found that 34% of Americans had used at least one unconventional therapy or remedy in the past year, and a third of these people visited unconventional therapists. More visits were made to providers of unconventional therapy than to all US primary care physicians. The expenditure on unconventional therapies ($13.7 billion) was comparable to that spent on all hospitalizations in the United States ($12.8 billion). Eisenberg *et al.* included vitamin and mineral supplements, and relaxation techniques in their definition of unconventional therapy so these results exaggerate the use of truly complementary therapies.

In Europe, surveys suggest that a third of people have seen a complementary therapist or used complementary remedies in any one year. The popularity of CM in Europe is growing rapidly. In 1981, 6.4% of the Dutch population attended a therapist or doctor providing CM, and this increased to 9.1% by 1985 and 15.7% in 1990. The use of homeopathy, the most popular form of complementary therapy in France, rose from 16% of the population in 1982 to 29% in 1987 and 36% in 1992 (Fisher and Ward 1994).

CM is generally used most often for chronic conditions such as musculoskeletal problems, arthritic conditions, respiratory disorders, skin conditions and psychological problems and sometimes for more serious conditions (Eisenberg, Kessler and Foster 1993; Thomas *et al.* 1991). High rates of use of CM have been found in patients with AIDS (Greenblatt *et al.* 1991; Hand 1989), arthritis and rheumatism (Boisset and Fitzcharles 1994; Visser, Peters and Rasker 1992), asthma (Donnelly, Spykerboer and Thong 1985) irritable bowel syndrome (Smart, Mayberry and Atkinson 1986) and cancer (Cassileth *et al.* 1984; McGinnis 1991). When CM treatments are used for serious conditions it is almost always as an adjunct to conventional treatment, rather than as a replacement for it. Doctors, counsellors and psychologists are likely to see a great number of patients using unconventional treatments, the majority of which will probably not be discussed with them. There is little indication that patients using CM have turned their backs on orthodox medicine, although they may have exhausted its possibilities in relation to a specific complaint (Eisenberg, Kessler and Foster 1993; Thomas *et al.* 1991). They are simply consumers in the health market.

PERSPECTIVES ON COMPLEMENTARY MEDICINE

Gray (1998) argues that 'the topic of unconventional therapies can no longer be ignored or marginalized because, for better or worse, each seriously ill person cannot help but be confronted with choices about their possible usage' (p. 55). He believes there are currently four quite different and debatable perspectives on complementary medicine:

(1) *The biomedicine perspective*   This is concerned with the curing of disease and control of symptoms where the physician-scientist is a technician applying high level skills to physiological problems.

> 'Biomedicine needs to be understood as a product of western culture, drawing on some of the dominant western philosophical traditions. Assumptions which thus permeate biomedicine include (1) that the natural order is autonomous from human consciousness, culture, morality, psychology and the supernatural; (2) that truth or reality resides in the accurate explanation of material (as opposed to spiritual, psychological or political) reality; (3) that the individual is the social unit of primary importance (as opposed to society); and (4) that a dualistic framework (e.g. mind/body) is most appropriate for describing reality.' (p. 57)

This approach is antagonistic toward and sceptical of CM, believing many claims to be fraudulent and many practitioners unscrupulous. Physicians and medical scientists within this camp often believe CM patients are naive, anxious and neurotic. However, the competitive health care market place has seen a shift even in the attitudes of 'hardliners' to being more interested in, and sympathetic to unconventional therapies.

(2) *The complementary perspective*   Though extremely varied, those with this perspective do share certain ideas such as (1) rating the importance of domains other than the physical for understanding health, (2) viewing diseases as symptomatic of underlying systemic problems, (3) a reliance on clinical experience to guide practice and (4) a cogent critique of the limits of the biomedical approach. Interventions at the psychological, social and spiritual level are all thought to be relevant and important supporting the idea of a biopsychosocial model. Many advocates of this perspective believe the body has powerful natural healing mechanisms that need to be activated. They are critical of biomedicine's harsh and often unsuccessful treatments, especially with cancer. They attack biomedicine for have most of its own interventions not being based on 'solid scientific evidence'.

(3) *The progressive perspective*   Proponents of this perspective are prepared to support either of the above, depending on the scientific evidence in

favour. They are hardened empiricists who believe it is possible to integrate the best of biomedicine and unconventional approaches. Like all other researchers, their approach is not value free—the advocates of this approach welcome the scientific testing of all sorts of unconventional therapies.

(4) *The postmodern perspective* This approach enjoys challenging those with absolute faith in science, reason and technology and deconstructing traditional ideas of progress. Followers are distrustful of, and cynical toward, science, medicine, the legal system and institutionalized religion and even parliamentary democracy. Postmodernists abandon all world views and see truth as a socially and politically constructed issue. Many believe orthodox practitioners to be totalitarian persecutors of unconventional medicine. They rejoice in, and welcome multiple perspectives and 'finding one's own voice'. However, because many CM practitioners can be theoretically convinced of their position and uncompromising, they can also be subject to postmodern scepticism. Proponents of this position argue (1) to have a complementary perspective in any debate is healthy, (2) that CM practitioners are also connected to particular economic and theoretical interests, (3) that the variety of values and criteria for assessing success is beneficial and (4) that the ill people themselves should be the final arbitrators of the success of the therapy.

Gray (1998) concludes:

'It has been argued above that both the biomedical and complementary perspectives tend to be characterized by strongly held beliefs about the nature of health, illness and reality, while the proponents of the progressive perspective subjugate such beliefs to the tests of scientific method, which in itself is characterized and influenced by values. Postmodernists argue that all perspectives are value-based and socially constructed, and that no one perspective will have all the truth about health practices, or anything else. They encourage the articulation of multiple perspectives as a basis for fully informed decision-making, with the individual ill person as final arbitrator.' (p. 70)

Gray's argument has a number of implications for this chapter and for understanding complementary medicine. First, the reader may wish to know that the authors' own perspective is, broadly speaking, progressive, tinged perhaps with biomedical sympathies. Second, it is important to be aware of the strongly conflicting beliefs and ideologies that come into play when complementary medicine is discussed. There are differences not only about what treatments are effective and what is valuable about complementary medicine, but at a more basic level about how these questions should be answered and, from the postmodern perspective, about whether they should be asked at all. Third, Gray's views highlight one of the principal dilemmas of complementary medicine, which is a debate about how it should progress. Should complementary practitioners align themselves with orthodox scientific medicine, or should they fight to preserve their own voice, perhaps even to the point of denying the validity of scientific attempts to validate or disconfirm complementary approaches? With these caveats in mind we turn to research into the efficacy of complementary medicine and other research-based explanations for its appeal.

PSYCHOLOGICAL AND SOCIOLOGICAL EXPLANATIONS FOR THE APPEAL OF COMPLEMENTARY MEDICINE

There is a mass of both anecdotal and carefully recorded evidence that patients of a wide range of complementary therapies benefit from the treatment. Clearly many patients 'feel better' after treatment: some are completely cured of their problem (migraine, back pain, smoking) while others report a 'decrease in pain, anxiety' etc. The problem for the research is accounting for that success. The central question is to what extent a therapy's success is a function of psychological or sociological mechanisms, discussed in this section, as opposed to the specific processes of the therapy, discussed below.

There is a rich, multi-disciplinary literature of the nature and function of health beliefs and how they operate. All adults have complex and interrelated ideas of wellness, illness and disease. They have been extensively exposed to folk theories, media stories and orthodox medical consultations which have shaped these ideas. Of course, demographic factors, such as social class, and individual difference factors, such as personality, also play a part in shaping, maintaining and changing health beliefs. Such beliefs underlie decisions to seek complementary treatment and may also underlie accounts of its success. Some have suggested, for instance, that reports of effective treatment may be attributable to *dissonance reduction* for payment or compliance with unpleasant treatments.

A more plausible explanation, however, is that CM practitioners do offer patients something genuinely beneficial and which ultimately does affect their health. The few studies of complementary consultations suggest that they contain elements that are particularly important to patients, who are more accustomed to a few minutes with a hard-pressed and overworked general practitioner (Vincent and Furnham 1997). Some elements of the consultation that are strongly emphasized in complementary consultations:

- Taking a full medical history that includes all aspects of the person's life-style, including beliefs, values, personal and work relationships. People have a holistic view of health, believing all aspects of their lives are interconnected. They expect any practitioner to take a history that allows the former to understand them as a person.
- Touching and examining the patient. The 'laying on of hands' has been forgotten in orthodox medicine but not counselling, where it has been revived. Patients expect to be examined, which helps build up the relationship with the doctor.

- Discussing the options, uncertainties, prognosis fully. Many, but not all, patients like to try to understand the cause of the problem, how the therapy works and their prognosis.
- Being more willing to consider, and to discuss, emotional problems and spiritual perspectives on health and illness.

These particular concerns about the consultation are one aspect of a more general dissatisfaction. The green and consumerist movements have led people to have quite different expectations about treatment. Practitioners of complementary medicine, if not orthodox medical doctors, have realized that patients want to be treated with respect—as adult customers. They resent crowded waiting rooms and being patronized. Educated middle-class patients, dissatisfied with orthodox consultations and treatment, are turning to various forms of complementary medicine to fulfil their needs. Patients want a consumer contract of equal responsibilities rather than allowing their doctors to feel entitled to make all the decisions about their health care.

More broadly, sociologists have argued that many patients have become disenchanted with orthodox medicine and its, to some, excessive reliance on high technology and loss of personal relationship between doctor and patient. There is a growing ambivalence about modern medical technology and advances and the media have put doctors and medicine on trial. There is now considerable fear of iatrogenic disease (problems that originate from medical intervention) and drugs which are supposed to cure, but only exacerbate the problem (Taylor 1985; Saks 1998). There has also been a medicalization of social issues and this always undermines people's own self-determination. Medicalization exercises both social control and surveillance over ordinary people's bodies and lives. Worse, the medicalizing individualism in the West has a victim-blaming ideology, which serves to transfer the burden of health costs from the state to the individual (Bakx 1991; Cant and Calnan 1991).

THE EFFICACY OF COMPLEMENTARY MEDICINE

We cannot, in a single chapter, hope to adequately review the evidence for the efficacy of complementary medicine. However, in considering the role of complementary medicine in health promotion, the evidence for its efficacy is fundamental. We therefore summarize the evidence for three of the major therapies—acupuncture, homeopathy and the manipulative therapies—concentrating on major reviews of randomized controlled trials. For a full account the reader is referred to Vincent and Furham (1997) and to the original review papers.

CM has often been chastised for the paucity of supportive evidence and the low standard of much of the evaluative work. Many studies of CM are indeed flawed by methodological problems. Poor design, inadequate measures and statistical analysis, lack of follow-up data and substandard treatment are all too common (Vincent 1993; Kleijnen 1991). However, deficiencies also abound in the orthodox medical literature (Williamson, Goldschmidt and Colton 1986; Sacks *et al.* 1987; Smith 1991). The quality of medical information generally, and in particular the evidence for many clinical interventions, is quite poor. The difference in the standards of evidence for orthodox and complementary therapies may not be as great as generally assumed.

While we, and most orthodox researchers, have accepted the validity of the double-blind, randomized control trial (RCT) many, even within orthodox medicine, have questioned the appropriateness of this 'gold standard' methodology. Difficulties in the evaluation of all treatments by RCTs include: (1) the blinding of subjects and/or clinicians not always being feasible; (2) participation in the study affecting behaviour and outcome; (3) nonrepresentativeness of trial subjects; (4) artificially standardized treatments; (5) inadequate attention to individual responses; (6) outcome measures that do not reflect the patient's concerns and (7) a variety of ethical issues (Kramer and Shapiro 1984; Pollock 1989; Grisso 1993; Lewith and Aldridge 1993; Pocock 1993; Vincent and Furnham 1997). In addition there are other concerns that are particular to complementary medicine. The major areas of concern are: (i) complementary theoretical frameworks, producing misunderstanding between conventional researchers and complementary practitioners; (ii) the use of unconventional diagnostic systems; (iii) problems with the blinding of trials; (iv) difficulties in defining an appropriate placebo control; (v) the insistence on individually tailored treatment, and individual measures of response; and (vi) the difficulty in finding outcome measures that reflect the particular perspective of complementary practitioners. These difficulties notwithstanding, however, it is possible to come to some broad, though provisional, conclusions about efficacy.

Acupuncture

Richardson and Vincent's (1986) review found good evidence for the short-term effectiveness of acupuncture for low-back pain, mixed results for headache, and some encouraging preliminary results for cervical pain and arthritis. The proportion of patients helped varied from study to study but commonly fell in the region 50–80%. In a later and larger review Ter Riet and colleagues (1990a) identified 51 controlled trials of acupuncture for chronic pain. Each study was scored on 18 methodological criteria, some weighted more heavily than others, with a maximum possible score of 100. Only 11 studies scored 50 or more points. Positive and negative results were approximately equally divided in the higher-quality studies. The treatment for musculo-skeletal problems of the spine (mostly low-back pain) showed the most positive results. Similar results are obtained when reviews are confined to studies with an acceptable placebo control (Vincent 1993). Inconsistent evidence of efficacy was found in a review of 13 controlled trials of acupuncture for asthma (Kleijnen, Ter Riet and Knipschild 1991a). Only three of fifteen studies of acupuncture for smoking showed a positive results and there was little evidence that acupuncture was of benefit in the treatment of heroin addiction (Ter Riet, Kleijnen and Knipschild 1990b).

Manipulative Therapies

Research on osteopathy and chiropractic therapies has, however, so far as randomized controlled trials are concerned, been largely limited to back and neck pain. Most trials compare a manipulative therapy with some simpler, cheaper therapy such as short-wave diathermy, massage and analgesics, though a few are comparisons of different manipulative techniques (Koes *et al*. 1991).

A number of reviews have been published, with broadly similar conclusions, but confidence in the standard of the studies appears to have slowly increased over the years (Greenland *et al*. 1980; Brunarski 1984; DiFabio 1986; Curtis 1988). The most comprehensive review of spinal manipulation (Koes *et al*. 1991) followed the same methods of the Kleijnen *et al*. (1991b) review of homeopathy. Thirty-five randomized controlled trials were identified, but no trial scored over 60 points out of a possible 100, though some of the standards are very difficult to attain. Thirty trials concerned the treatment of back pain, and five neck pain. In 18 trials (51%) the authors reported better results for spinal manipulation than for the comparison treatment, usually some form of basic standard treatment such as physiotherapy (short-wave diathermy, massage, exercises) or drugs (generally analgesics) or placebo. In 11 studies there was no difference between the spinal manipulation and the comparison treatment or the comparison was superior. Four of eight studies involving a placebo comparison, usually detuned short-wave diathermy, found a significant advantage for manipulation. Overall Koes and colleagues suggest that the results are promising, but not yet conclusive.

Homeopathy

The most comprehensive review of homeopathic treatment is by Kleijnen, Knipschild and Ter Riet (1991b), representing a herculean effort to track down all known controlled trials of homeopathy. A total of 107 controlled trials was identified, dealing with a variety of different conditions: diseases of the respiratory system (19 trials on respiratory infections, five on hay fever and one on asthma); 27 trials on pain of various kinds; gastrointestinal complaints (seven trials); diseases of the vascular system (nine trials, four on hypertension); recovery of bowel movements after surgery (seven trials); psychological problems (10 trials) and a variety of other diagnoses.

Overall, the findings were positive: of the 105 trials with interpretable results, 81 indicated positive results, and 24 trials had negative findings when homeopathy was compared with (mostly placebo) controls. The methodology of many of these trials is, however, quite poor, with 83 scoring 55 or below and only 16 scoring 60 or above. For instance, more than half the trials had fewer than 25 patients per group. Mindful of the fact that more positive findings can be associated with poorer methodology, the authors separated out the best studies, those scoring at least 60/100. Ten of the best studies show an advantage for homeopathy against four negative findings (and one which is inapplicable in that it was a comparison of homeopathic treatments).

Kleijnen and colleagues, who were initially extremely sceptical of the value of homeopathy, concluded that the evidence, although generally positive, was probably not sufficient for most people to form a definite view. They suggested that further large-scale trials, under rigorous double-blind conditions were definitely warranted. The discussion of the paper is thoughtful and especially interesting in the light of the authors own avowed scepticism about homeopathy. Their scepticism appears to have been at least dented, in that they conclude that 'we would be ready to accept that homeopathy can be efficacious, if only the mechanism of action were more plausible' (p. 321).

ADVERSE EFFECTS OF COMPLEMENTARY MEDICINE

Complementary therapies appear, on the limited evidence available, to be remarkably safe. Orthodox treatment is associated with a much higher level of risk, though clearly this must always be offset against the benefits of treatment for serious or life-threatening illness (Brennan *et al.* 1991; Einarson 1993; Vincent 1997). It has been argued that some therapies are dangerous (poisonous) but a more common criticism is that they can be no more than a commercial exploitation of the vulnerable to chronic or terminal illness (Vincent and Furnham 1997; Ernst, Siev-Ner and Gamus 1997). For some their danger lies most in giving hope to, or changing the expectations of, patients when it is inappropriate or judged retrospectively to be unhelpful.

Rampes and James (1995) reported a total of 216 instances of serious complications in acupuncture patients (such as pneumothorax) world-wide over a 20-year period, very low considering the large numbers of people receiving acupuncture. Infections from needles (mostly hepatitis) were the largest category, but are now of less concern as disposable needles are widely used. Patijn (1991) reviewed 93 cases of reports of complications during manual therapy, involving a total of 129 cases. In 16 cases of vertebral artery injury the patient died and in a further 55 there were permanent neurologic deficits. The actual rate of complications is impossible to ascertain, though it appears to be small as these appear to be the sum total of reported instances. There are almost no reports of direct adverse effects of homeopathy in the orthodox medical literature.

There have also been reports of harm coming to patients of complementary practitioners through their avoidance of beneficial, perhaps life-saving, orthodox treatment (Baum 1991). In fact very few patients of complementary practitioners have turned away from orthodox treatment (Thomas *et al.* 1991), though there may be a small number who eschew orthodox methods. Exactly how often this occurs and whether this is due to the influence of complementary practitioners is entirely unknown.

CULTIVATING HEALTH THROUGH COMPLEMENTARY MEDICINE

As must now be clear, there is no such thing as 'alternative' or 'complementary' medicine. Rather, there is a bewildering range of therapies ranging from the culture-specific to the more universal, from those primarily based on talk, or touch, or manipulation, to those relying on pharmacological changes. Some complementary therapies attempt to treat a small range of highly specific problems, i.e. back pain, while others believe their particular treatment will 'cure or successfully manage' a very wide array of mental and physical problems (depression, anxiety headaches, high blood pressure). Some practitioners have attempted to build alliances with orthodox medicine, while others are determined to maintain their separateness and autonomy. Some would like to join loose federations, others not. But most seek recognition and approval, not only by patients but also government bodies and funding agencies.

People in the West are increasingly educated and critical consumers of health care. For many, a consultation with a CM practitioner offers real help, be it relief from symptoms or psychological reassurance. Further, as educated consumers they are likely to use a variety of different specialists—both orthodox and unconventional—at the same time, while also self-medicating.

Patients consulting different types of complementary practitioners hold differing levels of scepticism about orthodox medicine. Patients differ by degrees in their health beliefs, and scepticism of orthodox medicine, and do not fall neatly into two distinct groups. It would also seem to be incorrect to talk of patients simply being 'pushed' or 'pulled' towards complementary therapies, as scepticism of the efficacy of orthodox medicine may be combined with greater concern for the planet, healthier life-styles, greater belief in the importance of state of mind, and more concern with the nature of the consultation. It is this combination, together with their particular medical history, that leads patients to consult complementary practitioners.

The attitudes to complementary medicine have also changed. While there have been vitriolic attacks on some aspects of CM (for example, Skrabanek 1988), many orthodox GPs appear to welcome links with complementary practitioners. Some are impressed by the evidence of efficacy while others, more pragmatically, see that any move towards self-care and a reduction in dependence on doctors might work in favour of orthodox medicine and overstretched health services. Any form of treatment that encourages people to become more health aware or to develop better coping strategies is obviously welcome. However, it seems unlikely that the costs of health care overall would be reduced because few complementary patients give up orthodox medicine.

Some, perhaps more cynical, orthodox medical practitioners embraced CM because they believe that unnecessary visits to GPs may be reduced. This is based partly on the rather cynical idea that many CM patients are chronic, psychosomatic cases that take up considerable amounts of GP time and show little response to orthodox treatment. Clinical and counselling psychologists attached to GP practices are also seen as a useful way of reducing the load and taking a difficult case whose prognosis is poor.

The line dividing orthodox and CM will always be changing. Some complementary therapies are probably destined always to remain outside conventional, scientifically based medicine. Others may gain acceptance and be no longer considered complementary, perhaps losing their unique character in the process. Acupuncture, for instance, is widely used in pain clinics, but not in its traditional form. The influence of CM, however, may be more pervasive and more important than any of its particular therapies. For many patients it represents a form of medicine that is more personal, less invasive and less risky, and which offers them more time and an opportunity to take an active part in their own treatment. Many current health problems are primarily problems of life-style that require a different kind of medicine. Conventional medicine may have to become more complementary in method and in spirit, while not relinquishing its scientific base and insistence on a critical evaluation of all forms of therapy.

APPENDIX: THE MAJOR COMPLEMENTARY THERAPIES

Acupuncture The human body is considered to be an energy system. The acupuncturist influences this energy flow by inserting and manipulating needles along the meridians of energy; restoring the balance of the energy flow restores health and harmony to the individual.

Herbalism Plants have been used for medicinal purposes for at least 5000 years. Herbal remedies can provoke protective reactions within the body, act to stimulate the elimination of toxins and provide the body with a balance of nutrients and minerals. Herbalists would consider that complex combinations of actual plant material are more effective than the specific isolated compounds used in modern pharmacology.

Homeopathy The homeopath stimulates the body's vital energies to prevent and treat disease. Diagnosis takes account of physical, emotional, mental and even moral factors. Homeopathic remedies would produce symptoms that are similar to those during treatment. They are frequently, but not always, diluted to the point where little, if any, of the original substance is left.

Manipulative therapies: osteopathy and chiropractic Osteopaths and chiropractors are skilled in the examination, treatment and interpretation of abnormalities of function of the musculo-skeletal system. They hold that many common conditions are caused, or at least aggravated, by misalignments or excessive strain placed on the vertebrae and other joints. They are primarily, but not exclusively, concerned with musculo-skeletal disorders.

REFERENCES

Bakx, K. (1991) The 'eclipse' of folk medicine in western society. *Sociology of Health and Illness*, 13.

Baum, M. (1991) Bridging the gulf. *Complementary Medical Research*, 5(3), 204–208.

BMA (1986) *Alternative Therapy*. Oxford: Oxford University Press.

Boisset, M. and Fitzcharles, M.-A. (1994) Alternative medicine use by rheumatology patients in a universal health care setting. *Journal of Rheumatology*, 21(1), 48–152.

Brennan, T.A., Leape, L.L., Laird, N.M., *et al.* (1991) Evidence of adverse events and negligence in hospitalized patients. *New England Journal of Medicine*, 324, 370–376.

Brunarski, D.J. (1984) Clinical trials of spinal manipulation: a critical appraisal and review of the literature. *Journal of Manipulative Physiological Therapy*, 7(4), 243–249.

Cant, S. and Calnan, M. (1991) On the margins of the medical market place? An exploratory study of alternative practitioners' perceptions. *Sociology of Health and Illness*, 13.

Cassileth, B.R., Lusk, E.J., Strouse, T.B. and Bodenheimer, B.J. (1984) Contemporary unorthodox treatments in cancer medicine. *Annals of Internal Medicine*, 101(1), 105–112.

Curtis, P. (1988) Spinal manipulation: does it work? *Occupational Medicine*, 3(1), 31–44.

DiFabio, R.P. (1986) Clinical assessment of manipulation and mobilization of the lumbar spine. *Physical Therapy*, 66, 51.

Donnelly, W.J., Spykerboer, J.E. and Thong, Y.H. (1985) Are patients who use alternative medicine dissatisfied with orthodox medicine? *Med. Jnl. Aust.*, 142(10), 539–541.

Downer, S.M., Cody, M.M., McLuskey, P. *et al.* (1994) Pursuit and practice of complementary therapies by cancer patients receiving conventional treatment. *British Medical Journal*, 309, 86–89.

Einarson, T.R. (1993) Drug-related hospital admissions. *The Annals of Pharmacotherapy*, 27, 832–840.

Eisenberg, D., Kessle,r R.C. and Foster, C. (1993) Unconventional medicine in the United States. *New England Journal of Medicine*, 328, 246–252.

Ernst, E. (1997) Integrating complementary medicine? *Journal for the Royal Society of Health*, 117, 285–286.

Ernst, E., Siev-Ner, I. and Gamus, D. (1997). Complementary medicine—a critical review. *Israel Journal of Medical Sciences*, 33, 808–815.

Fisher, P. and Ward, A. (1994) Complementary medicine in Europe. *British Medical Journal*, 309, 107–111.

Fulder, S.J. and Munro, R.E. (1985) Complementary medicine in the United Kingdom: patients, practitioners, and consultations. *Lancet*, 2(8454), 542–545.

Gray, R. (1998) Four perspectives on unconventional therapy. *Health*, 2, 55–74.

Greenblatt, R.M., Hollander, H., McMaster, J.R. and Henke, C.J. (1991) Polypharmacy among patients attending an AIDS clinic: utilization of prescribed, unorthodox, and investigational treatments. *Journal of Acquired Immune Deficiency Syndrome*, 4(2), 136–143.

Greenland, S., Reisbord, L.S., Haldeman, S. and Buerger, A.A. (1980) Controlled clinical trials of manipulation: a review and a proposal. *Journal of Occupational Medicine*, 22, 670.

Grisso, J.A. (1993) Making comparisons. *Lancet*, 342(8746), 157–160.

Hand, R. (1989) Alternative therapies used by patients with AIDS. *New England Journal of Medicine*, 320(10), 672–673.

Kleijnen, J., Ter Riet, G. and Knipschild, P. (1991a) Acupuncture and asthma: a review of controlled trials. *Thorax*, 46(11), 799–802.

Kleijnen, J., Knipschild, P. and Ter Riet, G. (1991b) Clinical trials of homeopathy. *British Medical Journal*, 302, 316–323.

Koes, B.W., Assendelft, W.J.J, van der Heijden, G.J.M.G., Bouter, L.M. and Knipschild, P.G. (1991) Spinal manipulation and mobilisation for back and neck pain: a blinded review. *British Medical Journal*, 303, 1298–1303.

Kramer, M.S. and Shapiro, S.H. (1984) Scientific challenges in the application of randomized trials. *Journal of the American Medical Association*, 252(19), 2739–2745.

Lewith, G.T. and Aldridge, D. (1993) *Clinical Research Methodology for Complementary Therapies*. London: Hodder & Stoughton.

McGinnis, L.S. (1991) Alternative therapies 1990. An overview. *Cancer*, 67(6 Suppl), 1788–1792.

Patijn, J. (1991) Complications in manual medicine: a review of the literature. *Journal of Manual Medicine*, 6, 89–92.

Pocock, S.J. (1993) *Clinical Trials*. Chichester: Wiley.

Pollock, A.V. (1989) The rise and fall of the random controlled trial in surgery. *Theoretical Surgery*, 4, 163–170.

Rampes, H., James, R. (1995) Complications of acupuncture. *Acupuncture in Medicine*, 13(1), 26–33.

Richardson, P.H. and Vincent, C.A. (1986) Acupuncture for the treatment of pain: a review of evaluative research. *Pain*, 24, 15–40.

Sacks, H.S., Berrier, J., Reitman, D. and Ancona, B.V.A. (1987) Meta-analyses of randomized controlled trials. *New England Journal of Medicine*, 316(8), 450–455.

Saks, M. (1998) Medicine and complementary medicine: Challenges and change. In E. Scambler and P. Higgs (Eds) *Modernity, Medicine and Health*. London: Routledge.

Skrabanek, P. (1988) Paranormal health claims. *Experientia*, 44(4), 303–309.

Smart, H.L., Mayberry, J.F. and Atkinson, M. (1986) Alternative medicine consultations and remedies in patients with the irritable bowel syndrome. *Gut*, 27, 826–828.

Smith, R. (1991) Where is the wisdom . . .? *British Medical Journal*, 303(6806), 798–799.

Taylor, R. (1985) Alternative medicine and the medical encounter in Britain and the United States. In: J. Salmon and P. Warren (Eds) *Alternative Medicine* (pp. 191–235). London: Tavistock.

Ter Riet, G., Kleijnen, J. and Knipschild, P. (1990a) Acupuncture and chronic pain: a criteria based meta-analysis. *Journal of Clinical Epidemiology*, 11, 1191–1199.

Ter Riet, G., Kleijnen. J. and Knipschild, P.A. (1990b) Meta-analysis of studies into the effect of acupuncture on addiction. *British Journal of General Practice*, 40, 379–382.

Thomas, K.J., Carr, J., Westlake, L. and Williams, B.T. (1991) Use of non-orthodox and conventional health care in Great Britain. *British Medical Journal*, 302(6770), 207–210.

Vincent, C.A. (1993) Acupuncture as a treatment for chronic pain. In: G.T. Lewith and D. Aldridge (Eds) *Clinical Research Methodology* (289–308). London: Hodder and Stoughton.

Vincent, C. and Furnham, A. (1996) Why do patients turn to complementary medicine? An empirical study. *British Journal of Clinical Psychology*, 35, 37–48.

Vincent, C. and Furnham, A. (1997) The perceived efficacy of complementary and orthodox medicine: a replication. *Complementary Therapies in Medicine*, 5, 85–89.

Vincent, C., Furnham, A. and Willsmore, M. (1995) The perceived efficacy of complementary and orthodox medicine in complementary and general practice patients. *Health Education Research*, 10, 395–405.

Visser, G.J., Peters, L. and Rasker, J.J. (1992) Rheumatologists and their patients who seek alternative care: An agreement to disagree. *British Journal of Rheumatology*, 1, 485–490.

Williamson, J.W., Goldschmidt, P.G. and Colton, T. (1986) The quality oi medical literature: an analysis of validation assessments. In J.C. Bautar and R. Mostellar (Eds) *Medical Use of Statistics* (pp. 370–391). Waltham, MA: NEJM Books.

Chapter 8

Boiled Nettles in May: Studies of Plural Medicine in Northern and Southern Ireland

Anne MacFarlane* and Pauline Ginnety

This chapter addresses medical pluralism and its relevance for health promotion. Medical pluralism occurs where different medical systems, with different underlying philosophies, compete and jostle with each other at any given time (Stainton-Rogers 1991). In the past, several different medical systems existed in society on largely equal terms but, with the growth of science, biomedical medicine became privileged and the other forms were, at best, not recognised or, worse, treated by biomedicine as 'quackery'. Contemporary research shows that rather than disappear, many of these systems are still in existence and utilised by people as explanatory models and as aids to treatment (e.g. Helman 1978). Furthermore, systems of folk medicine from other traditions are being drawn upon by increasing numbers of people in Western society (Sharma 1995). Biomedicine (or allopathic medicine) still remains privileged in that it is the dominant form of 'official' medicine in our society while the other forms mostly remain outside of the mainstream health services as private or voluntary activities undertaken by individuals.

The purpose of this chapter is to explicate the relevance of medical pluralism and folk health knowledge to health promotion. We will draw on the reality of people's beliefs and behaviours about and for health. We will focus particularly on the range of responses people can, and do, make in the face

Cultivating Health: Cultural Perspectives on Promoting Health. Edited by M. MacLachlan.
© 2001 John Wiley & Sons Ltd.
* formerly Murphy.

of illness. When confronted by a symptom people do not usually rush to their doctor. They go through a process of reflection during which they draw on their own health knowledge (which will include a combination of folk, traditional, alternative and bio-medical concepts) and act according to what they feel is appropriate and/or accessible to them.

Such diversity in health-seeking behaviour—medical pluralism—provides a positive perspective from which to view people's broad-ranging health practices. This has implications for health promotion because if people draw on a wider body of knowledge to explain and act on symptoms it is likely that they will consult that same body of knowledge when deciding on preventive or protective courses of action.

CASE STUDY

SEARCHING FOR RELIEF*

Mike Barry is a painter and decorator. While he is busy most of the time he occasionally experiences gaps between jobs and these are financially worrying for himself and his family. On a recent job, he experienced a sudden pain in his back and was shocked when he realised that he had 'slipped a disc'. The pain was very severe and made it impossible for him to work. His wife, Mary, was very concerned about him as were his extended family. They all tried to help in some way, asking their friends for advice. Mary talked a lot to her mother Pat about the situation and they both watched Mike's progress carefully. In particular, they considered the various treatment options he had tried.

> Mary: 'I don't know, Mam, poor Mike, he's in an awful way with this slipped disc. He was at the chiropractor, you know? Oh, it was terrible and he had a bomb spent on him. So he went to a bonesetter there last week. They are supposed to be gifted people, you know. Marvellous people.'
> Pat: 'But Mary, why on earth did he go off to see a chiropractor and bonesetter? What about the doctor? I mean what is a chiropractor anyway? There was nothing like that in my day!'
> Mary: 'Oh God! his back was very bad. It really was very bad. And he did go to the hospital first. That day he went into the hospital, they gave him an X-ray and they said they'd put him in traction.'
> Pat: 'But was it the doctor told him to go to the chiropractor?'
> Mary: 'Oh no, no. A friend of mine had been there before and she had great success with this chiropractor and had been telling me all about it. So Mike went to the chiropractor, he had to do something you know, the pain was so bad. He got a massage there. Now, it was very expensive. It cost him a bomb, you know. Thirty pounds a session I think he said it was. I suppose he had to try it though, didn't he?'
> Pat: 'But did that massaging do him any good? After spending all that money!'
> Mary: 'Well then his back seized up altogether, it was locked. So the chiropractor said he couldn't do any more for him. And then someone else advised the

* This case study is based on material gathered in an interview conducted in Cork city, Southern Ireland, October 1995 (MacFarlane 1998a).

bonesetter. That was the idea some other friend had. You probably know all about bonesetters do you?'

Pat: 'I do! Funny isn't it, I remember the bonesetter from when I was young. My two brothers were up to the bonesetter a few times with sprained ankles and broken bones and so on. I hadn't heard much talk of bonesetters these past years at all.'

Mary: 'Well, Mike headed down there last week. In the meantime, he has an appointment with some specialist, you know, but he'll have to wait another four or five months for that.'

Pat: 'Was the bonesetter any good?'

Mary: 'I think so. It was tough enough though. He told me that it was very excruciating, very severe. Seemingly the bonesetter was only £12, you know, so that's quite good isn't it? So, he went through that treatment that day and has definitely been less locked up, less painful. He's wondering now what the specialist can do for him as well, that will be the next thing.'

Pat: 'And what did the doctors in the hospital have to say about this treatment from the chiropractor and the bonesetter?'

Mary: 'Well, I don't know now to be honest. But Mike . . . well he was in an awful situation and he was just left waiting all that time for his appointment with that specialist. He had to try something you know. He was worried, sure we were all worried. At least he was able to try those other treatments. They had worked for other people so, you know, he had the choice, to feel he was able to do something, not just wait and wait. But, I suppose, no, he didn't say anything now to those doctors, because, well, they mightn't like that kind of thing. They might give out or think you were a bit mad. I mean, that's fine but . . . Mike was in such pain.'

SCALING UP

The outcome of Mike Barry's search for relief is not known. However, his story illustrates the varied and diverse ways in which people behave with respect to their health, that is their health-seeking behaviour. This represents an area of major importance for the health-promotion movement. It is important to understand the factors and processes involved in health-seeking behaviour as they reflect both individual and community/societal beliefs about health maintenance, disease prevention and responses to illness. Thus, they can be important in the development of health-promotion programmes.

A review of the body of work on health promotion in Western societies reveals that socio-psychological models are often employed including the health locus of control model (e.g. Goldsteen, Connte and Goldsteen 1994) and the health belief model (e.g. Becker and Maiman 1974). Such approaches have three main limitations. First, these models are overly individualistic. Second, most health-seeking behaviour research has tended to be excessively quantitative in terms of methodology (see e.g. Stainton-Rogers 1991). Third, the biomedical focus of research on health-seeking behaviour in Western societies is problematic since biomedicine is '. . . a healing system which is based upon a biological understanding of the human being and stresses these aspects above others' (Currer and Stacey 1986: 3).

To take each of these limitations separately, the first point about individualised approaches being applied to societies, has been well developed by the Research Unit in Health and Behavioural Change (RUHBC 1987) who argue that in the 1940s the public health movement in Britain 'picked up the wrong end of the social science stick' and chose an individual rather than socio-cultural approach resulting in micro (individual) soluations being applied to macro (community) health problems.

The second limitation referred to a predominance of quantitative research approaches being used in health-promotion research and activity. The utilisation of large-scale surveys tends to be the dominant approach in biomedical or public health research and tends to reflect the concerns of the researcher rather than the researched. While this approach may be appropriate to biomedicine, we would argue that it is less appropriate for health promotion since the focus of the research may fail to address the concerns of the community or client group. Such methods provide aggregate data which demonstrate associations between demographic variables and aspects of physical and mental health and illness. However, they do not explain how such variables interact at individual, family, community levels nor how health may be understood as one component of daily life (Macintyre 1986). Furthermore, in claiming to be 'value free', the research approach may not uncover the alternative perceptions of health held by different societies or social groups. Qualitative research methodologies, on the other hand, start with the individual or group, and are firmly rooted in the social context. In recent years a number of studies by sociologists have addressed the issue of health and illness from the perspective of people themselves (Blaxter 1990; Cornwell 1984; Graham 1985, Herzlich 1973).

The third point, about the biomedical focus of research on health-seeking behaviour, is related to the reasons for undertaking such research. Very often, the rationale for much of the research on health-seeking behaviour has stemmed from perceived problems with health service usage and concerns about 'inappropriate' illness behaviour by patients. Professional perceptions of 'appropriate' illness behaviour tended to be associated with compliance with biomedical advice in terms of service utilisation and adherence to treatment (Mechanic 1989). 'Inappropriate' utilisation of health services has been viewed from the medical perspective as non-compliant or deviant behaviour which required correction (see Morgan, Calnan and Manning 1985). 'Deviance' of this kind might be seen as visiting the GP with a unnecessary minor problem such as a cold; failing to recognise the need for medical services for more serious symptoms relying on treatment at home involving old remedies or self-care treatments or visiting a acupuncturist or chiropractor with a recurring back problem. However, if the social, cultural and historical context of these health-seeking behaviours were recognised by those working in health care then such behaviours could be intrepreted as resourceful or functional behaviour. Levin, Katz and Holst (1979) have discussed this in relation to self-care practices. They argue that health professionals' perceptions of self-care are negative and have an emphasis on replacing redundant health practices while simultaneously enhancing compliance with modern medicine.

There is ample ethnographic evidence demonstrating that people draw upon non-biomedical ideas (see Cornwell 1984) and use non-biomedical practices (Sharma 1995). Despite this, the full range of responses to illness which have been documented in research using, for example, health diaries (Verbrugge and Ascione 1987 in Freund and Maguire 1995) has been largely ignored by those researching health-seeking behaviour, as well as those working in the health-promotion field. While some quantitative work has been conducted in this area (see Chapter 7), few qualitative studies have been undertaken on heath-seeking behaviour in Western societies, with the notable exception of Ursula Sharma's (1995) study of complementary medicine in Britain.

In order to clarify some of the terms used in this chapter a brief descriptive account of several forms of health-seeking behaviours will now be given.

Self-care

Self-care has been described as the most predominant and basic form of primary care (Padula 1992) and also constitutes the largest system of health care (Helman 1978). It is an historical and universal form of health care (Haug, Wykle and Namazi 1989) embracing disease prevention, diagnosis, treatment and long-term management of health and illness (Padula 1992). Self-care practices may include eating a healthy diet, the use of nutrition supplements, keeping clean and warm, taking regular exercise, bed-rest and utilisation of over-the-counter-medication (Spector 1991). Traditional home remedies, derived from folk medicine, may also constitute self-care practices. The maintenance of knowledge and the intergenerational transmission of information about folk medical self-care practices is considered by Lipson and Steiger (1996) with particular reference to the role of women as health workers and healers. Such folk remedies and ideas have often been dismissed as 'old wives' tales'. Yet scientific research has demonstrated the efficacy of some traditional remedies, their medicinal properties have been accepted within the scientific corpus of knowledge and, as O'Suilleabhain (1994) argues, used or developed in modern medical practice. The remedy cited as the title for this chapter, for instance, refers to the use of boiled nettles in spring as a means of cleansing the blood and ensuring good health. The iron content within nettles would, of course, explain the reasoning and wisdom within this folk remedy. The contribution that folk knowledge makes to research by the pharmaceutical industry is too often ignored or downplayed. A lack of regulations regarding patenting means that 'foreign' scientists are in a position to commercialise and claim ownership of traditional medicines that have been used for centuries by local healers (Agarwal and Narain 1996).

Traditional healers

Healing refers to the beneficial influence of a person on another living thing by mechanisms which are beyond those recognised and accepted by conventional medicine (Benor 1984). Such healing has been recorded in all parts of the world, with earliest references from China, India, Assyria, Egypt (Meek 1977, in Benor 1984), and generally involves the laying on of hands and/or prayer and meditation. Various explanations have been proposed for these healing mechanisms. Some healers believe that they stimulate internal innate healing forces within the person, while other suggestions refer to a transfer of healing energies from the healer to the healee. It has also been proposed that the role of the healer is as an intervention channel between spiritual forces and the patient (Benor 1984). There is considerable heterogeneity among healers. In South Africa, for instance, *inyangas* use herbal treatments for healing purposes, *isangomas* are diviners using ancestral spirits and *umthandazi* are Christian faith healers (Kane 1995).

ALTERNATIVE AND COMPLEMENTARY MEDICINE

Attempts to define alternative medicine are generally unhelpful because they try to categorise vastly heterogeneous groups of treatments and practices collectively (Pietroni 1992). The result is often a 'list' rather than a conceptual defintion (Taylor 1984). Fulder (1986) argues that non-conventional medical systems in Western societies are in fact traditional or indigenous healing systems from other parts of the world. He describes these common origins quite specifically and, in doing so, identifies links between traditional folk remedies, folk healers, alternative practitioners and biomedicine:

> 'Complementary medicine today is a descendant of traditional and folk medicine: herbalism from shamanism and folk remedies, chiropractic and osteopathy from bone setting, homoepathy from early like-cures-like principles, naturopathy form the Hippocratic lineage. Curiously, scientific medicine traces its origins to those same roots, via Galen of Pergamum in the 2nd century A.D.' (Fulder 1986: 237)

It has been argued that trying to evaluate the effectiveness of complementary therapies are fraught with practical (Tonkin 1987) and methodological difficulties (see Lewith and Alderidge 1993). However, some positive scientific evidence has been found for acupuncture (e.g. Meade *et al*. 1991). Even if we do not know exactly how treatments work, recent experience in Western societies, as well as more historical experience in non-Western countries, indicates that some therapies do produce a desired effect of enhanced health and well-being.

In recent times, awareness of the co-existence and competition between biomedicine and complementary medicine has increased. Studies throughout Western countries, for instance, the United Kingdom (Thomas, Carr, Westlake and Williams 1991), the United States (Eisenberg *et al*. 1993), Europe (Sermeus 1987) and Australia (Lloyd, Lupton, Wiesner and Hasleton 1993) have documented utilisation rates for various forms of complementary treatments. A general finding has been that people from middle to higher income groups are among those most likely to report use of complementary medicine. Although chronic illnesses tend to feature strongly, a wide range of different conditions have been cited by people who use complementary medicine.

Dissatisfaction with biomedicine has been identified frequently as a key motivating factor underlying people's reasons for turning to complementary treatments (e.g. Sharma 1995; Murray and Rubel 1993; Fulder 1988) and particularly difficulties with the practitioner/patient relationship (see Taylor 1984). However, there is also strong evidence that people who choose to use some form of complementary medicine are not abandoning biomedicine entirely. Concurrent use of both medical systems has been recorded in Britain (Thomas, Carr, Westlake and Williams 1991) and Canada (Northcott and Bachynsky 1993). This is consistent with findings from studies undertaken in non-Western societies.

The exploration of the different ways in which people respond to illness experiences and, moreover, the implications of such diversity for 'co-existing' and 'competing' types of medicine is enhanced by taking an historical perspective. While the emphasis in research on plural medicine in Western societies has tended to focus on decisions to visit a non-biomedical practitioner, such as complementary therapists, less attention has been paid to the contact people may have with traditional folk healers. Although it has been proposed that folk healers have been replaced by different and more exotic practitioners (see Skrabanek 1994), the persistence of traditional forms of healing and understanding of health and illness in industrial and non-industrial societies (Helman 1978; Kleinman 1984) suggests that they meet a need. Thus, it is necessary to acknowledge heterogeneity within plural medicine (Young 1983). Recent research undertaken in both Northern and Southern Ireland has approached the study of plural medicine from this more heterogeneous perspective. Specifically, old and new forms of heterodox medicines have been examined. This chapter compares and contrasts findings from these databases.

IRISH RESEARCH

This section begins with a brief descriptive account of some recent research undertaken by the authors in Northern and Southern Ireland, all of which employed qualitative methodologies. Figure 8.1 shows the locations of these four Irish studies.

Details of the research findings will then be presented. Insights from these findings, and implications for health promotion practice, will conclude the chapter.

In 1992, the Eastern Health and Social Service Board (EHSSB) in Northern Ireland initiated an ethnographic study of health-seeking behaviour with the Travelling community in Belfast (Ginnety 1993). Travelling people represent a separate ethnic group in Irish society with a distinct culture defined by

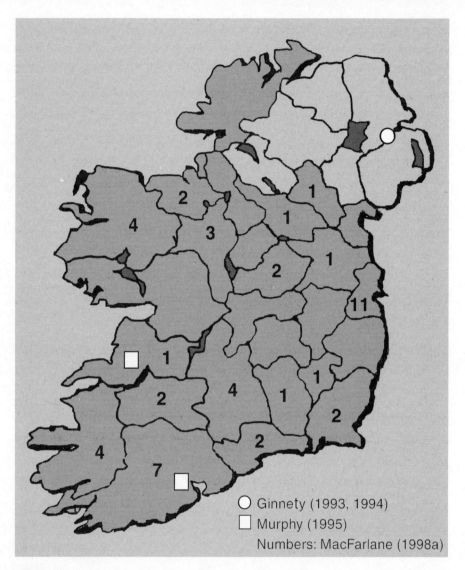

Figure 8.1   Map of areas where data were collected

self-ascription as Travellers, a shared history, shared customs and traditions, including nomadism and a shared language. Their needs had largely been ignored in health-care planning and health service provision prior to the 1990s. Travellers' poor health status and low life expectancy* represents an example of the Inverse Care Law as described by Tudor-Hart (1971) by which those with fewer health needs consume more of the available services

---

* Barry, Herity and Solan (1989) demonstrated high standardised mortality ratios in Travellers relative to the general population. For example, SMRs for Traveller women were 307 compared to 140 for women from social class 5 in the settled population. Traveller men's SMRs were 222 compared to 150 for settled men in social class 5.

than those with greater needs. Following a period of getting to know members of the Travelling families who were living in Belfast by attending social events, such as weddings and funerals, the researcher was in a position to be sufficently accepted to begin interviewing. Altogether a total of 55 in-depth interviews were undertaken with both male and female Travellers. Their experiences with formal biomedical health services and complementary systems of healing were explored.

The material gathered from the 'Health of Travellers' study was compared with the documented experiences of members of a settled community (Ginnety 1994). This was another qualitative study conducted with 50 participants over a 9-month period in a working-class area of Belfast. Of these, 43 were women who, as the primary carers for their families, had much experience of health and illness. Participant observation and informal interviewing methods were used.

Meanwhile in Southern Ireland, two studies of plural medicine were instigated by the Department of Health Promotion, National University of Ireland, Galway. The first of these, conducted in 1993–1994, was a cross-sectional qualitative study (Murphy 1995). It was a replication of a 1930s folklore study, which employed children's essays as a means of collecting information in a rural area on the west coast of Ireland as well as in an urban area in the south. The aim was to document the relative prevalence of biomedicine, traditional folk medicine and complementary medicine in contemporary Ireland. In total, 519 children's essays entitled 'Health Practices' were collected through 21 primary schools. In keeping with the original methodology, material for the essays was gathered from older family and community members by the children as part of a homework exercise. These essays were analysed in terms of reported health knowledge and reported use of each type of medicine.

The second study involved a national interview study (MacFarlane 1998a). Participants for this research were drawn from an existing database of older people in Ireland aged 65 years and over. This had been developed by the Economic and Social Research Institute, Dublin, for the purposes of a National Council for the Elderly survey of the health and autonomy of Irish older people (Fahey and Murray 1994).

A 'piggy-back' survey was arranged whereby those within the ESRI database between the ages of 69 and 72 years were invited, using postal survey methods, to participate in the national interview study. Fifty-one in-depth interviews were conducted in 22 counties. The number of participants interviewed in each county is shown in Figure 8.1 illustrating the geographical spread of the study. The interest in meeting with older people within this specific age range relates to the fact that, by virtue of their age, some would be original participants of the 1930s folklore study. This was considered important because associations between different kinds of non-biomedical practices had been recorded in the children's essay study outlined above (Murphy and Kelleher 1995). Similarly, Sharma (1995) had found some links between childhood use of traditional folk medicine and a later interest in using complementary medicine. Thus, the extent to which childhood involvement with, or exposure to, traditional folk medicine might influence interest in 'new' alternatives to biomedicine was of particular interest. In summary, the aim of these interviews was to explore patterns of biomedical and nonbiomedical health-seeking behaviour throughout the lives of the older people with particular reference to changes over time.

Irish Research Findings

Descriptions of traditional Irish folk medicine were obtained in the studies cited above. These descriptions included details of herbal remedies and magico-religious cures as categorised by Yoder (1972). Herbs and plants were prepared within the home for the purposes of maintaining health; garlic was considered effective for preventing colds and 'flu. As referred to earlier, preparing soup with nettles in the spring or summer was described as a preventive treatment to cleanse the blood and, thus, promote good health: '. . . it used to clear your blood, a feed of nettles . . . once a year. In the spring of the year they'd tell you . . . the nettles, the green nettles that we'd pick and put them into a saucepan and boil them for soup' (quotes from MacFarlane 1998a).

Other references to herbs and plants pertained to treating illnesses; a mixture of boiled milk, onions and pepper was considered a good treatment for colds. The extent to which household materials were utilised was also evident as the use of bedsheets for preparing bread poultices to treat boils was described. Stockings full of salt were tied around the neck of someone suffering from a sore throat. The relevance of ritualistic features from the magic–religious category of folk medicine, such as the role of boundaries and ideas about transference are evident in the following description of a cure for warts from the 1930s children's essay folklore archive:

> 'Count the warts, get as many small pebbles and put them in a piece of cloth and leave it at the cross-roads. Whoever found it and counted the pebbles it is they would get the warts—and they would go out of the person that would have them. . . .'

The role of women as health workers was noted in both the Northern and Southern Irish studies. For instance, the responsibility placed on women for informal health care was noted within the settled community in Belfast (Ginnety 1994). Similarly, MacFarlane (1998b) explored the transmission of folk medical knowledge over time and found that references to knowledge being passed on 'from generation to generation' was most likely to mean female family members recounting knowledge and passing practical skills to each other.

The kind of traditional healers that people in the Southern studies were familiar with included bonesetters, seventh sons of seventh sons, someone whose father had died before his/her birth, a woman who married a man of the same surname (i.e. if a McCarthy married a McCarthy) and, finally, faith healers (Murphy and Kelleher 1995). Beliefs about the acquisition of skills varied although healing power from God was common to seventh sons of seventh sons as well as faith healers. Some faith healers described had clerical backgrounds, such as priests or canons, while others did not. The following comment is from an older man in the Travelling community in Northern Ireland: 'I don't believe much in curing men and women, I believe in clergymen' (Ginnety 1993: 94). However, overall in the Northern Irish studies there was less reference to the origins of the healer's gift or skill but rather to the outcome of the activity (Ginnety 1993).

Associations between the nature of presenting symptoms and the use of traditional folk remedies or traditional healers was evident in both datasets (Ginnety 1993; Murphy 1995). For instance, the kind of ailments for which folk remedies were cited were predominately skin conditions and musculoskeletal problems (Murphy 1995).

The extent to which folk remedies and traditional healers were used currently in Northern and Southern Ireland was explored. It was apparent that there was a considerable amount of knowledge about traditional medicine among all participants to the extent that details of remedies and practices, as described above, could be provided. This knowledge base was found to be particularly strong in the rural area studied in Southern Ireland whereby descriptive details of folk medicine were provided in 95% of the children's essays (Murphy and Kelleher 1995). There was also considerable evidence that people nowadays were less inclined to acknowledge use of such folk remedies. Less than a quarter of the participants from the rural children's essay survey reported that they or their family would use traditional medicine currently. Similarly, older people interviewed throughout Southern Ireland said that they would sometimes use certain remedies or treatments currently but the dominant view was that folk medicine had been used more so in the past, that it had been useful but its time had passed. Interestingly, despite these views, participants were quite critical or, at times, offended at the idea that younger people would laugh at traditional folk medicine. One man commented sadly that younger people today would tell you to 'go and dance' if you mentioned a cure or remedy. (MacFarlane, 1998).

These findings echo the views of participants from both the settled and Travelling community in Northern Ireland. While the urban settled dwellers 'laughed' at the idea of older self-care practices, a few hinted that as they themselves approached middle age they were more inclined towards remedies used by their mothers. This could be due to their increasing life experience and a scepticism about biomedicine. Some spoke of antibiotics and antidepressants being prescribed 'too freely' by local doctors. Similarly, most of the Travelling people who spoke about spiritual forms of healing were in the middle to older age range. Very few young people mentioned these options. However, a particular form of spiritual healing mentioned by the urban settled people was the application of St Anne's oil. This was used by women themselves as an adjunct to biomedical treatment. They applied it for a variety of physical ailments including breast lumps.

There is some evidence from the children's essay survey that those from lower socio-economic backgrounds may be more likely to use traditional folk medicine currently. Conversely, use of complementary medicine was found to be more likely among those from higher non-manual backgrounds (MacFarlane and Kelleher 1997). Acupuncture, herbalism, reflexology and homeopathy were the types of complementary therapies used. The cost of complementary treatments was cited specifically as the main deterrent to their use by some urban dwellers from low-income backgrounds in Belfast. An interest in acupuncture as a treatment or method for quitting smoking was thwarted by the financial cost of treatment.

There were no accounts of the Travellers in Northern Ireland using complementary medicine. This may reflect financial costs as a barrier to treatment but also the context in which complementary medicine is offered. In Northern Ireland, complementary medicine tends to be provided in settings which require particular social networks which may be closed to Travellers. Indeed, the relative ease of access to biomedical health services for settled people with higher incomes has perhaps allowed them to dispense with traditional forms of medicine and to experiment with other new alternatives. This may not be the case for members of the Travelling community in Northern Ireland whose access to formal health care was seen to be more limited and problematic (Ginnety 1994). This interpretation reflects Sharma's (1995) view that contemporary exploration and practice of alternative medical viewpoints might be born out of choice rather than necessity, which was the case for previous generations.

Older people in Southern Ireland were shown to be very cautious about using complementary medicine and, indeed, few of them had. These participants generally indicated a strong reliance on their GP for health advice. Socio-cultural factors were cited as explanations for these changing patterns of health-seeking behaviour in terms of having a broad knowledge base about treatments as well as being influenced by 'customary' practices (MacFarlane 1998). An interesting issue within this comparative analysis is the role played by people's 'lay referral networks' as described by Freidson (1961). It is known that health-seeking behaviour is informed by the ideas and experiences shared within people's lay referral networks. This means that people rely on their own social contacts for advice on care and on possible suitable forms of treatment. If it is not customary for people within a particular network to seek treatment from a given source, for whatever reason (e.g. financial and social constraints have been cited above), then it is not within the 'pool' of ideas and experiences for sharing, which in turn does not encourage use. This might explain the fact that accounts of contact with complementary practitioners are so minimal among the older people and Travelling people in our Irish studies. This would concur with Berger and Luckmann's (1966) argument that although knowledge is transmitted from generation to generation (by language) not everybody possesses the same knowledge. This refers to the social distribution of knowledge along lines of gender, social class, age, ethnicity and division of labour.

INSIGHTS

A number of themes emerge from the material presented above, and these have relevance for health promotion. They include the role of women in the transmission of health knowledge from generation to generation, the notion of 'lay competence' in health, and the socio-cultural context of health-seeking behaviour.

Women as Health Workers

The health work conducted by women over time, across medical systems and across different social and cultural groups has been highlighted in recent Irish research. This corresponds with Lipson and Steiger's (1996: 7) view that:

> 'Women have always been healers . . . For centuries women were doctors without degrees, barred from books and lectures, learning from each other, and passing on experiences from neighbour to neighbour, and mother to daughter. They were called "wise women" by the people, witches or charlatans by the authorities.'

The other constant feature in this area is the 'taken for granted' nature of women's roles in the health arena. This has been explained by Gavron (1966) and Oakley (1974), among others, in relation to social and cultural assumptions about women and femininity. Consequently, women's work is 'hidden' and operates in the private domain whereas biomedicine which, until recently, was predominantly a male preserve, is privileged and operates in the public sphere.

Lay Competence

The description of plural medicine in Ireland provided above has highlighted the existence of a range of non-biomedical treatments and practices. The use of such treatments has been discussed in relation to various issues including the socio-economic environment and the nature of presenting conditions. It is argued here that all these data point to the pragmatic nature of health-seeking behaviour. It has been shown in this chapter that people address an illness experience with questions such as, 'How serious is this?' 'What kind of treatment or medicine is available?' 'What have other people used in this situation?' 'What were the outcomes?' The essential drive behind such questioning is, of course, a desire to be better. The disruptiveness of illness to people's lives cannot be underestimated. It is this perspective on pluralistic responses to illness that Sharma (1995) has emphasised in her qualitative study of complementary medical use in Britain. Sharma (1995) argues strongly that searching for a 'type' of complementary medical user may be misguided. Again and again in her interviews, people from diverse and varied background and situations emphasised the pragmatism behind their practices—they just wanted to be well and re-engage in social and economic activity:

> 'An exhausted actress, a depressed youth leader, a saleswoman with psoriasis—for these people actual or impending failure to meet the quotidian demands of a job prompted the move from orthodox to non-orthodox treatment when the pace of progress was felt to be unsatisfactory.' (Sharma 1995: 40)

It is, perhaps, this very pragmatism that informs pluralistic responses to illness and, moreover, leads to *dynamism* in pluralism. We have seen that the kind of alternatives available to people and, indeed, considered acceptable to people in Ireland changes over time. This is not, of course, peculiar to Ireland. Lambert (1996) has emphasised the universality of dynamism within health-seeking behaviour in Rajasthani in Northern India. She writes that:

> 'Rajasthani villagers, like people world-wide, are willing and eager to adopt new technologies that work and to change their health-seeking behaviour and preferences accordingly.' (Lambert 1996: 348)

Medical pluralism may also reflect a desire for autonomy. People can 'dip into' non-biomedical forms of care and maintain control. As Sharma shows, this is rarely the case with biomedical care where 'doctor's orders' still prevail.

Socio-cultural Context of Health-seeking Behaviour

No apparent link was found between people's level of contact with traditional folk medicine and their use of non-indigenous traditional medicines among either members of the Travelling community or older people in Ireland. On the one hand, this is surprising as associations between different kinds of non-biomedical practices had been recorded previously (e.g. Murphy and Kelleher 1995; Sharma 1995). However, on the other hand, these findings might reflect the impact of cultural preferences for treatment; people's level of access to alternative forms of medicine, as well as the social distribution of knowledge between generations (Berger and Luckmann 1966).

RECOMMENDATIONS

The central recommendation to be made, following research on medical pluralism in Northern and Southern Ireland, is for the adoption of a collaborative approach between health workers and the people with whom they work. For some years, arguments for a shift from authoritarian approaches to more collaborative approaches have been articulated both within and without the biomedical domain (WHO 1978). There has been a recent call for biomedical practitioners to have more respect for the 'brains and imaginations of patients, more development of patients as critical observers, measurers, and recorders of their own illnesses' (Tudor-Hart 1997). This is important as it recognises that practitioners and patients act as co-producers of health.

With respect to specific initiatives to promote health, collaboration and participation between practitioners and the people with whom they work is, of course, of paramount importance. Increasingly, the appropriateness and, indeed, the value of a community development approach is being recognised within health promotion work. Labonte (1998) and others have demonstrated the relevance of community development to health promotion. This approach recognises that in order to improve the health of communities, their needs must be known and the people themselves must be to the forefront in identifying them and in proposing the solutions for addressing them.

In Northern Ireland, official recognition was given to the community development approach and its relevance for health when it was incorporated into the 1997–2002 Regional Strategy for Health and Social Services (Department of Health and Social Services (DHSS) 1996). This recognition allows those involved in health promotion to extend the boundaries of their work. A range of initiatives has resulted at many levels ranging from the regional level through to communities themselves. For example, the Community Development and Health Network Northern Ireland has taken the opportunity afforded by the DHSS policy to embed community development approaches in existing structures, through a 'Policy to Practice' initiative (Community Development Health Network Northern Ireland 1998). At Board level, the Eastern Health and Social Services Board initiated a Health Perceptions Project in four communities in Belfast. Local people participated in identifying their own community's health needs and brought them to the attention of health authorities. Moreover, the local people continue to participate with health workers in taking action to bring about change (Eastern Health and Social Services Board 1998). Voluntary and community groups also demonstrate the importance of community development approaches to their work in the promotion of health (Barnardo's 1998; Creggan Health Information Programme 1997). Although some of these developments have emerged from structures committed to a biomedical approach, they give recognition to other ways of looking at health rather than through lenses that are exclusively biomedical. Most important of all is that some statutory organisations recognise the need for structural change is emanating from a 'lay' model. In Southern Ireland there is, to date, no formalised commitment to community development within health promotion. However, there is a strong tradition of community development work in the South, particularly in relation to social and economic issues. Also, some recent research concerning the health needs of rural communities has moved toward a

community development approach with the formation of partnerships between community members and health board representatives (Barry *et al.*
1998, submitted).

The benefits of collaboration and dialogue between health practitioners
and the people with whom they work are multiple. Encouraging dialogue
between practitioners and patients, using a systematic review of patients'
preferences, values and needs, has been described by Delbanco (1992) with
explicit reference to the issue of plural responses to illness:

> 'When patients choose acupuncture, massage, guided imagery, folk healing or
> homeopathy, how do we respond if our experiences or values conflict? Patients
> who are encouraged and invited to do so can tell us more about 'non-
> traditional' therapies they embrace. In turn, we can care for them in a less
> judgmental way as we learn how they understand and approach their own
> health and disease.' (Delbanco 1992: 416)

Such an approach would also resolve existing ambiguous norms around
perceptions of 'appropriate' passivity and activity in patients' roles as
considered by Freund and McGuire (1987). This approach is also consistent
with the ethos of health promotion as an empowering and participative
concept. Consider the benefits of shared decision making through dialogue
between practitioners and patients. Patients could be involved in a real
way, bringing their own experiences and observations into play as well as
enhancing their existing knowledge base of a particular health matter leading to further empowerment. Moreover, such collaborative approaches to
decision making in health care would demonstrate 'official' acknowledgement for the competent way in which people approach health matters and
illness experiences.

A second recommendation relates to the extent to which people draw on
plural ideas and practices about, and for, health. This has implications for
health promotion in terms of people's beliefs and practices about preventing
illness and maintaining health. Thus, within the dialogic processes recommended previously, care must be taken to consider the range of diverse
sources from which people draw their ideas about health and illness.
Theories of disease causation held by lay people are strongly influenced by
both personal experiences and observations of the experiences of others (e.g.
Blaxter and Paterson 1982) as well as cultural or spiritual beliefs (e.g. Ager *et
al.* 1996). The need to pay particular attention to culture as a dimension of
health has been well argued by Airhihenbuwa (1995) who has emphasised a
need for health workers to understand the relevance of culture in all societies. Ethnocentric tendencies have been noted within Western perspectives, particularly in relation to multiculturalism in health-care management
and delivery (e.g. MacLachlan 1997).

This final point, regarding multiculturalism and health, requires special
consideration within the Irish context. Unlike countries such as the United
States, Canada and Britain, Southern and Northern Ireland are often thought
to be considerably less multi-cultural. This view is problematic because it does
not acknowledge the extent to which the Travelling community in Ireland

represents a distinct and separate ethnic group and, for example, the consequent implications for health services delivery and health-promotion initiatives. Also, this view is incompatible with the reality that people from varied cultural backgrounds do live throughout Ireland (Central Statistics Office 1996). It is also worth considering the extent to which Ireland will become *more* multicultural in future years as indicated by current patterns of asylum seeking in Ireland (personal communication, One World Centre, Galway, Ireland).

IMPLICATIONS

The implications of these recommendations can be illustrated with reference to our case study of Mike Barry's search for relief. The functional nature of Mike's health-seeking behaviour and the careful way in which possible options for treatment were reflected upon by Mike and his extended family provides a live example of diversity and pluralism in day-to-day health care. As recommended in the previous section, it would have been most beneficial if the biomedical practitioners involved in Mike's care had provided an opportunity for him to share his ideas about other possible treatments for his slipped disc. The use of a patient's review (Delbanco 1992) would have been useful for this purpose. Such dialogue between biomedical health workers would have produced a participative environment in which Mike could have actively engaged in the consultation sessions. Moreover, he could have shared his knowledge about other people's experiences with chiropractors and bonesetters for treating back problems. A non-judgmental view of the diverse way in which Mike had approached his situation would have been beneficial in two regards. First, it would have been respectful of the care taken in making these health decisions. Second, it would have acknowledged that non-biomedical forms of treatment can provide effective treatment options for people. This kind of acknowledgement is, of course, deserved and represents a rich opportunity for learning for all health workers. Also, a collaborative consultation would have meant that Mike would not have felt any reluctance or hesitation around discussing his treatment choices openly. Rather, the various choices open to him could have been experienced in an empowering manner only.

These implications have focused only on the context of doctor/patient consultations. In essence, these reflect a health-promotion approach within health-care delivery. However, as discussed in our recommendations, there are implications for all health workers, particularly those involved in health-promotion initiatives in terms of the 'status' awarded to the 'lay' people with whom they work. Collaboration has benefits for all parties involved. The extent to which non-biomedical ideas have informed health care has been raised in this chapter with respect to the common origins of plural medical systems (Fulder 1986) as well as the development of natural substances in modern pharmacology. Indeed, it is from such sharing that we have learned, among many other things, the benefits of boiling nettles in May.

REFERENCES

Agarwal, A. and Narain, S. (1996) Pirates in the garden of India. *New Scientist*, October.

Ager, A., Carr, S.C., MacLachlan, M. and Kaneka-Chilongo, B. (1996) Perceptions of tropical health risks in Mgonda, Malawi: Attributions of cause, suggested means of risk reduction and preferred treatment. *Psychology and Health*, 12, 23–31.

Airhihenbuwa, C.O. (1996) *Health and Culture: Beyond the Western Paradigm*. Thousand Oaks, CA: Sage.

Barnardo's (1998) *An Evaluation of the Chinese Lay Health Project*. Northern Ireland: Barnardo's.

Barry, J., Herity, J. and Solan, J. (1989) *The Traveller Health Status Study: Vital Statistics of Travelling People, 1987*. Dublin: Health Research Board.

Barry, M.M., Hope, A., Doherty, A. and Kelleher, C. (1998) Evaluation of mental health promotion programmes for rural communities. Paper presented at the Ninth European Symposium of the Association of European Psychologists, Beaunse, France.

Barry, M.M., Doherty, A. Hope, A., Kelleher, C. and Sixsmith, J. (submitted) A community needs assessment for rural mental health promotion.

Becker, M.H. and Maiman, L.A. (1974) Socio-behavioural determinants of compliance with health and medical care recommendations. *Medical Care*, 13, 10–24.

Benor, D.J. (1984) Psychic healing. In J.W. Salmon (Ed) *Alternative Medicines: Popular and Policy Perspectives*. London: Tavistock.

Berger, P. and Luckmann, T. (1966) *The Social Construction of Reality*. London: Allen Lane.

Blaxter, M. (1990) *Health and Lifestyles*. London: Tavistock/Routledge.

Blaxter, M. and Paterson, E. (1982) *Mothers and Daughters: A Three-Generational Study of Health Attributes and Behaviour*. London: Heinemann.

Central Statistics Office (1996) *Census 1996*. Dublin: CSO.

Community Development and Health Network Northern Ireland (1998) *Policy to Practice in Community Development*. Newry: CDHNI.

Cornwell, J. (1984) *Hard Earned Lives: Accounts of Health and Illness from East London*. London: Tavistock.

Creggan Health Information Programme (1997) *Children of Creggan Report*. Derry: CHIP.

Currer, C.S. and Stacey, M. (Eds) (1986) *Concepts of Health, Illness and Disease*. Oxford: Berg.

Delbanco, T.L. (1992) Enriching the doctor–patient relationship by inviting the patient's perspective. *American College of Physicians*, 116(5), 414–418.

Department of Health and Social Services (1996) *Health and Well-being: into the Millenium*. Belfast: DHSS:

Eisenberg, D.M., Kessler, R.C., Foster, C., Norlock, F.E., Calkins, D.R. and Delbanco, T.L. (1993) Unconventional medicine in the United States. *The New England Journal of Medicine*. 328(4), 246–252.

Fahey, T. and Murray, P. (1994) *Health and Autonomy among Over-65s in Ireland*. Dublin: Economic and Social Research Institute.

Freidson, E. (1961) *Patients' View of Medical Practice*. New York: Russell Sage Foundation.

Freund, P.E.S. and McGuire, M.B. (1995) *Health, Illness and the Social Body: A Critical Sociology*. Englewood Cliffs, NJ: Prentice Hall.

Fulder, S. (1986) A new interest in complementary (alternative) medicine: towards pluralism in medicine? *Impact of Science on Society*, 36(3), 235–242.

Gavron, H. (1966) *The Captive Wife*. Harmondsworth: Penguin Books.

Ginnety, P. (1993) *The Health of Travellers*. Belfast: Eastern Health and Social Services Board.

Ginnety, P. (1994) A cross cultural study of folk health knowledge. PhD thesis, Queen's University, Belfast.

Goldsteen, R.L., Counte, M.A. and Goldsteen, K. (1994) Examining the relationship between health locus of control and the use of medical services. *Journal of Ageing and Health*, 6(3), 314–335.

Graham, H. (1985) Providers, negotiators mediators: women as the hidden carers. In Lewin and Olesen (Eds) *Women, Health and Healing*. London: Tavistock.

Hand, W.D. (1971–1973) Folk curing: The magical component. bealoideas. *The Journal of the Folklore of Ireland Society*, 39–41, 140–156.

Haug, M.R., Wykle, M.L. and Namazi, K.H. (1989) Selfcare among older adults. *Social Science and Medicine*, 29(2), 171–183.

Helman, C.G. (1978) 'Feed a cold and starve a fever'. Folk models of infection in an English suburban community and their relation to medical treatment. *Culture, Medicine and Psychiatry*, 2, 107–137.

Herzlich, C. (1973) *Health and Illness: Social Psychological Analysis*. New York and London: Academic Press.

Kane, R. (1995) Traditional healers in South Africa: A parallel health care system. *British Medical Journal*, 310, 1182–1185.

Kleinman, A. (1984) Indigenous healing systems of healing: questions for professional, popular and folk care. In J.W. Salmon (Ed). *Alternative Medicines: Popular and Policy Perspectives*. London: Tavistock.

Labonte, R. (1998) Community development approaches. Background paper for Scottish Health Education Group/Research Unit in Health and Behavioural Change, Edinburgh.

Lambert, H. (1996) Popular therapeutics and medical preferences in rural north India. *The Lancet*, 348, 1706–1709.

Levin, L.S., Katz, A. and Holst, E. (1979) *Self-care: Lay Initiatives in Health*. New York: Provost.

Lewith, G.T. and Alderidge, D. (1993) *Clinical Research Methodology for Complementary Therapy*. London: Hodder and Stoughton.

Lipson, J.G. and Steiger, N.J. (1996) Self-Care Nursing in a Multicultural Context. Thousand Oaks, CA: Sage.

Lloyd, P., Lupton, D. and Hasleton, S. (1993) Choosing alternative therapy: an exploratory study of sociodemographic characteristics and motives of patients resident in Sydney. *Australian Journal of Public Health*, 17(2), 135–145.

MacFarlane, A. (1998a) Medical pluralism in Ireland 1930s-1990s. PhD thesis, National University of Ireland, Galway.

MacFarlane, A. (1998b) The changing role of women as health workers in Ireland, *Women Studies Review, Volume Five: Women and Health*. Galway: Women's Studies Centre.

MacFarlane, A. and Kelleher, C. (1997) Contemporary health practices in Ireland: manual versus non-manual differences (letter). *Irish Medical Journal*, 90(6), 240.

MacIntyre, S. (1986) The patterning of health by social position in contemporary Britain: Directions for social research. *Social Science and Medicine*, 23(4), 393–415.

MacLachlan, M. (1997) *Culture and Health*. Chichester: Wiley.

MacLachlan M. and Carr, S. (1994) From dissonance to tolerance: Toward managing health in tropical countries. *Psychology and Developing Societies*, 6(2), 119–129.

Morgan, M., Calnan, M. and Manning, N. (1985) *Sociological Approaches to Health and Medicine*. London: Croom Helm.

Murphy, A. (1995) Contemporary health practices in Ireland: an urban/rural analysis, MA thesis, National University of Ireland, Galway.

Murphy, A. and Kelleher. C. (1995) Contemporary health practices in the Burren, Co. Clare. *Irish Journal of Psychology*, 16(1), 38–51.

Murray, R.H. and Rubel, A.J. (1992) Physicians and healers—unwitting partners in health care. *New England Journal of Medicine*, 326(1), 61–64.

Northcott, H.C. and Bachynsky, J.A. (1993) Concurrent utilisation of chiropractic, prescription medicines, non-prescriptions medicines and alternative health care. *Social Science and Medicine*, 37(3), 431–435.

Oakley, A. (1974) *The Sociology of Housework*. Oxford: Martin Robertson.

One World Centre *Asylum Seekers, 1992–1998*. Galway. Personal communication.

O'Suilleabhain, S. (1994) In P. Logan (Ed) *Irish Folkcures*. New York: Sterling Publishing.

Padula, C.A. (1992) Selfcare and the elderly: Review and implications. *Public Health Nursing*, 9(1), 22–28.

Pietroni, P.C. (1992) Beyond the boundaries: relationship between general practice and complementary medicine. *British Medical Journal*, 305, 564–566.

Pope, C. and Mays, P. (1995) Reaching the part other methods cannot reach: an introduction to qualitative methods in health care research. *British Medical Journal*, 311, 42–25.

Research Unit in Health and Behavioural Change (1987) *Changing the Public Health*. Chichester: Wiley.

Sermeus, G. (1987) *Alternative Medicine in Europe. A Quantitative Comparison of the Use and Knowledge of Alternative Medicine and Patient Profiles in Nine European Countries*. Brussels: Belgian Consumers' Association.

Sharma, U. (1995) *Complementary Medicine Today: Practitioners and Patients.* London: Routledge.

Skrabanek, P. (1994) Irish traditional medicine: the foxglove ordeal and other folk 'cures'. *The Irish Colleges of Physicians and Surgeons*, 23(4), 121–126.

Spector, R.E. (1991) *Cultural Diversity in Health and Illness.* Connecticut: Appleton and Lange.

Stainton-Rogers, W. (1991) *Explaining Health and Illness: An Exploration of Diversity.* Hertfordshire: Harvester Wheatsheaf.

Taylor, R.C.R. (1984) Alternative medicine and the medical encounter in Britain and the United States. In J.W. Salmon (Ed.) *Alternative Medicines: Popular and Policy Perspectives.* London: Tavistock.

Thomas, K., Carr, J., Westlake, B. (1991) Use of non-orthodox and conventional health care in Great Britain. *British Medical Journal*, 302(26), 207–210.

Tonkin, R.D. (1987) The role of research in the rapprochment between conventional medicine and complementary therapies: discussion paper. *Journal of the Royal Society of Medicine*, 80, 361–363.

Tudor-Hart, J. (1971) The inverse care law. *The Lancet*, 405–412.

Tudor-Hart, J.T. (1997) What evidence is there for evidence based medicine? *Journal of Epidemiology and Community Health*, 51(6), 623–629.

Williams, R. (1983) Concepts of health: An analysis of lay logic. *Sociology*, 17(2), 185–205.

Yoder, D. (1972) Folk medicine. In R. Dorson (Ed.) *Folklore and Folklife.* Chicago: University of Chicago Press.

Young, A. (1983) The relevance of traditional medical cultures to modern primary health care. *Social Science and Medicine*, 17(16), 1205–1211.

Part III

SPECIAL ISSUES IN CULTIVATING HEALTH

Chapter 9

Traditional Mechanisms for Cultivating Health in Africa

Karl Peltzer

CASE STUDY

Clients consult traditional healers in Malawi for a variety of social problems, including economic and occupational problems, family problems, sorcery, witchcraft, and theft, and security and legal problems.

Mr Mandala lives in a major city in Malawi. He had finished secondary school and wished to start a business. His brother gave him money to start the business, and for a successful beginning he consulted a traditional healer. He was given herbal powder, for which he paid 30 Kwacha as a deposit of 150 Kwacha (at that time Kw5 was equal to £1), and took the powder to the place where he wanted to set up his business. Inside the house he said the following prayer (originally in Chichewa):

> 'Lord I beg you, give me luck in my business.
> There is no one else who can give me luck for business apart from you.
> And remove the darkness on my business.
> There is no one else who can remove darkness from business apart from you.'

In addition, he was advised by the healer that the business 'medicine' would only work if he and his wife followed these rules: love your father and mother and God; do not commit adultery; do not drink beer; and love your neighbour as you love yourself. The 'medicine' for prosperous business was *Desmondium velutinum* (*chinyambata*), *Erythrorylum emarginatum* (*mulungamo*), *luni-bayo* and *mbalachanda* leaves, pounded and made into a ball, together with some

Cultivating Health: Cultural Perspectives on Promoting Health. Edited by M. MacLachlan.
© 2001 John Wiley & Sons Ltd.

oil. The ball is smoked on burning *lubani*, tied into a cloth and put into the pocket (where the money is kept).

Chinyambata leaves stick to clothes, so that, symbolically, customers stick to the business. The word 'mulungamo' comes from 'chilungamo', meaning justice, which he should practice in his business, with the help of God's power. *Mbalachanda* is believed to attract customers. *Lubani* is an incense that should please the ancestral spirits so that they make customers visit the supplicant's enterprise. After some time, when Mr Mandala was not making progress in his business, he returned to the traditional healer. He was given another 'medicine' to try, but again returned after three months of unsuccessful business.

Mr Mandala felt that he could not prosper because of his uncle, who is against both him and his father. His father is the best and most modern farmer in the village. His yields are very high because he applies fertilizer. His uncle does not apply fetilizer and thus has only poor yields. Consequently he is jealous of his brother and also of his brother's son (Mr Mandala), who wanted to become rich quickly.

To start the business Mr Mandala's brother gave him 250 Kwacha. His borther is a carpenter and he advised him to buy fish for 160 Kwacha. He also sought advice from some people who knew the fish business. When selling the fish he felt he was making enough money, but when he arrived home he found that he made a loss. Indeed be believed that his uncle had magically taken some of the money. Thereafter he tried his luck with vegetables, but with the same outcome.

Although Mr Mandala says he followed all the instructions he was given by the healer, and that he administered the 'medicine' properly, his business enterprise still failed. He does not believe that he was given the wrong herbs, because he has heard of so many people who have been helped by Bwanali (the traditional healer). He is sure that it is his uncle's fault. However, after a lengthly interview with Mr Mandala one may question whether it is the fault of his uncle, since miscalculations with the money seemed to have led to his losses (Peltzer 1987).

This case study clearly illustrates both the powerful belief in, and realistic constraints on, the efficacy of traditional methods of problem solving in Africa. We now review the wide range of interventions that may be used to cultivate health and well-being in traditional African contexts.

INDIGENOUS METHODS

Indigenous Methods of Preventive Community Healing

Katz and Wexler (1989) describe community healing among the Kalahari *!Kung*. The primary ritual among the *!Kung*, the all-night healing dance, epitomizes the characteristics of sharing and egalitarianism. In the crucible of intense emotions and the search for protection which is the healing dance, sharing and egalitarianism are put to the test, relied upon as vehicles for survival. The healing power, or *n/um*, is the most valued resource at the dance, and one of the most valued resources in all community life. It is released by the community and, through its healing effects, helps to recreate and renew the community. Sometimes, as often as four times in a month, the women sit around the fire, singing and rhythmically clapping as night falls, signaling the start of the healing dance.

The entire camp participates. The men, sometimes joined by the women, dance around the singers. As the dance intensifies, *n/um* ('energy') is activated in those who are healers, most of whom are among the dancing men. As *n/um* intensifies in the healers, they experience *!kia* ('a form of enhanced consciousness') during which they heal everyone at the dance. Through *!kia*, the *!Kung* transcend ordinary life and can contact the realm of the gods and the spirits of dead ancestors. The dance provides healing in the most generic sense: it may cure a sick body or mind as the healer pulls out sickness with a laying on of hands; mend the social fabric as the dance promotes social cohesion and a manageable release of hostility; protect the camp from misfortune as the healer pleads with the gods for relief from the Kalahari's harshness.

These integrated functions of the dance reinforce each other, providing a continuous source of curing, counsel, protection and enhancement. To heal depends upon developing a desire to 'drink *n/um*', not on learning a set of specific techniques. Teaching focuses upon helping students overcome their fear, helping them to regulate the boiling *n/um* and resultant *!kia* so that healing can occur. The *n/um* must be hot enough to evoke *!kia*, but not so hot that it provokes debilitating fear. Accepting boiling energy for oneself is a difficult process because *n/um*, painful and mysterious, is greatly feared.

Tsala Tsala (1998) reports on the *mevungu* rites as a traditional form of group psychotherapy for women in Cameroon. The *mevungu* rite appears as an initiation rite with social function linked to femininity. It is repeated and ordered by men whenever the society is experiencing problems with regard to fertility issues. An all-night ritual is performed with women involving dancing, incantations, possession, and fertility procedures. The author suggests that women's cultural, political and professional associations in urban Cameroon have similar functions and objectives as *mevungu*, in the form of celebrations involving songs, dances, alcohol consumption, and licentious statements.

Indigenous Methods in Dealing with Death as a Prevention of Illness

One form of prevention from spirit illness which has similarities to the dance and song therapy of *vimbuza* (spirit illness) is the 'big dance' (*gule wamkulu*), practised during funeral ceremonies in central Malawi. During the funeral *gule wamkulu* (the male dancers who wear specific masks) perform before a mainly female audience who understand that the dancers are animals. The community tries to overcome its grief following the death of important members through a dramatic performance. Thus the spirit of the deceased should be settled properly and hindered from coming back and attacking individuals in the form of bad dreams or illness.

The symbolic meaning of the 'dancing animal' should be explained. According to the secret society the animal's foundation or origin is the bamboo (*nkonoto*). Bamboos grow in water and water means life. When the *gule wamkulu* member asks in their secret language 'where does the animal (*nyau*) hibernate when the water is full and when the water is dry?' the symbolic meaning of 'water is full' is 'many people' and 'water is dry' is few people. The answers to these two questions are as follows. When 'water is full' it is above the knees, and in the latter case it is at the feet or on the ground. The knees and level of the feet symbolically indicate that the more people in a society, the happier the animal (which here represents the *mzimu* or spirits of departed ancestors) becomes, and the lower the level of water (symbolizing the dying rate of the population). This makes the animal sad, which explains why it falls to the ground. In this context the water gives life to bamboos, which symbolize people. Without bamboos there are no people. Symbolically new life (the bamboo) has come from the seas, just as the new life of a baby come from water or amniotic fluid. Now when the animal dances it represents the resurrection of the deceased person into newborn life. The *nyau* (animal) eats soil (*ntoto*) which means in the secret language the water in which the *nyau* takes its bath. Symbolically the soil is left when someone dies and the water gives new life (Peltzer 1987).

Another form of dealing with death as a prevention of illness is found in the occurrence of victims of war or other forms of violence in Africa. In this context of 'unnatural' death the person may have disappeared or the corpse may not be found. Traditional and spiritual healing techniques concerning disappearance and death may involve: confirmation that is still alive (divination), confirmation of death (divination), rituals to bring the spirit of the dead home, symbolic burial (e.g. of fruit) in the absence of a corpse, and ritual appeasement of an afflicted family member:

(1) *Divination for whether the person is alive or dead*   A Madi traditional healer from Sudan may throw the cowry shells six to eight times and also consults the ancestral spirits. As a result, it will be confirmed whether the person who had disappeared is alive or dead. If it is confirmed that the person is alive then the patient will be reassured by the spirits not to worry and that their person will eventually come. If the person is dead, three stages may be followed. In the first the patient is prepared for the bad news: he or she is told that there is another problem which is coming soon, observing the patient's reaction, and then the patient may be told to come back another time so that he or she can communicate with the (dead) person. During the second stage the

patient is told about the death of their relative. Sometimes the patient comes back and finds that his or her relative must have died. Then the cowry shells are thrown to confirm that the person has died and consoling words are uttered to the patient (the money given for the deposit is returned). On returning home the patient must write a message for the deceased and burn it together with some herbs. At the third stage the relatives of the buried person consult the traditional healer in order to discover the cause of the death (e.g. curse from elders, disagreements/ envy, spirits were not brought home by elders).

(2) *Rituals to bring home the spirit of the dead*   A Madi healer from Sudan reports that first a hut has to be erected for the deceased. Then both the paternal and maternal relatives have to be present including the uncle of the deceased. A male goat has to be slaughtered and part of the meat (the hind legs) is kept hanging overnight in the hut meant for the deceased. Finally, the maternal uncles of the deceased have to say some protective words to avoid this happening.

(3) *Symbolic burial*   In the absence of the corpse and if no bones of the deceased can be discovered a traditional burial with a fruit called *Nyumburi* is conducted. The *Nyumburi* fruit symbolises the bones or corpse of the deceased closing the gate of death. It is just like a lock ending the whole matter about death and bringing a blessing to the well-being of family members. During the day of the funeral rites the *Nyumburi* fruit is buried in the traditional way that corpses are buried. A fireplace is set, uncles are given their cigarettes, and the previous ash of the fireplace collected and thrown away. The family consultation may take place as follows. People related to the unburied person come to discover whether there are any problems with the deceased person, e.g. incomplete marriage (agreed bride price not yet paid) or problems with ancestors. After these consultations agreements are made about shortfalls to be addressed, a prayer is held, and a burial of the *Nyumburi* fruit is conducted (Peltzer 1996).

Dreams, Stories, and Proverbs as Indigenous Psychohygienic Messages

Interpretations of dreams, the narration of stories, and proverbs are associated among the Yoruba in Nigeria with the elders, not only because they may have more experience and wisdom but also because it is in their interest to maintain the existing structure of their society. Psychologically, dreams, stories, and proverbs refer to an authority dimension, embodied in the elders and ancestors. Children learn through education and imitation of respected elders how to behave towards other people in the framework of a hierarchy, e.g. by recognizing oneself in allegorical terms in dreams, stories, metaphors, and proverbs one is able to establish self-confidence, trust and security. Dreams, stories, and proverbs give direct access to a human being by learning from oral tradition, and help to identify with and participate in human behaviour, decisions, and conflicts.

Considering the significant communicative role of dreams, stories, and proverbs in the everyday behaviour and socialization processes in Nigeria, then specific utilization for psychohygienic purposes becomes evident (for example, dreams of 'a message from a deceased relative' or 'food' or 'sex'). A message from a deceased relative is usually seen as advice to protect the children, or it may be in the form of a warning. For example: 'A man dreamt about his brother who had died long ago. In the dream his brother told him the cause of his death. He said that his brother told him to be aware of wicked people because they are planning to kill him too. The dream became true in the sense that some people are planning to eliminate him in the village.'

Food and sex dreams, as well as dreams of swimming, are believed to cause illness. It was reported that eating in dreams was very dangerous because one could easily be poisoned. The type of food that one could not eat in the dreams were kolanuts, meat, cooked food, fish and some fruits such as mango, orange, paw-paw and plantain. For example: 'I ate with strangers in my dream and on the following day I got abdominal pains . . . only God saved me.' Another example of this theme is: 'I had a dream that someone was eating in my house as a result of a ceremony which took place in my compound on that day. After some days the man who had eaten the rice developed serious abdominal pain, and he was taken to the hospital where he finally died.' Sex dreams are believed to cause impotence in males and infertility in females (Peltzer 1990).

Banks (1998) refers to storytelling as useful for learning more about historical and contextual factors affecting the well-being of women of African descent. Bührmann (1984) found that dreams among the Nguni in South Africa have the following functions: (1) to untreated, afflicted persons dreams serve as pointers indicating how they should seek assistance; (2) during the *vumisa* ('to diagnose by divination') they can have a diagnostic significance; (3) during treatment they indicate the various steps to be taken and their correct timing of; (4) they have a therapeutic value; and (5) they also have a prognostic value.

Indigenous Family Planning

Obisesan *et al.* (1997) studied family planning aspects of the practice of traditional healers in Ibadan, Nigeria. Cultural beliefs associated with fertility by traditional healers were that 37% agreed that 'People should have at least as many children as their parents did' and 31% 'If a couple have no male child, they should keep having more children in order to produce a male child'. Their perceptions of ideal child spacing is most commonly 2–3 years, which is consistent with the traditional belief that post-partum sexual abstinence should last for at least two years, and also that of World Health Organisation recommendations. While most of them recommend traditional methods of contraception (such as beads 70%, rings 68%, herbs 54%, abstinence during periods 48%, withdrawal 40%, chewing stick 25%) to their clients, up to 22% recommend modern family planning methods such as condoms (22%) and oral contraceptive pills (13%). Nearly all (95%) think that traditional healers and Western doctors should cooperate to provide family planning services

Indigenous Faith Healing Treatments for Substance Abuse, Chronic Diseases, and Protection from Witchcraft

Table 9.1 gives a summary of some faith-healing methods in South Africa. The indigenous faith-healing principles of purification, the use of tea, coffee or salt, confession, behavioural techniques, and proscriptions are outlined below.

Table 9.1 Methods of faith healing for alcohol abuse, 'high blood pressure' and protection from witchcraft

Alcohol abuse
Prayer, confession, baptism
Emetics
Antabuse
Inhaling, drinking
Bible reading
Water, tea, salt, ashes, herbs
Ashes, herbs, blessed beer
Blessed coffee, tea, holy papers, holy water
Proverbs to guide an alcoholic

High blood pressure
Prayer
Diet
Holy water
Blood letting
Medical check-up
Reduce: fat, salt, sugar; increase: milk, eggs, carbohydrates
Washing the body, inhaling holy steam
Nose cavities are punctured to get rid of 'bad blood'
Referral is made

Protection from witchcraft
House
Cars
Body
Nails, stones, or ashes are buried at four corners of the yard
Protective objects are tied or put into the car
Holy wool is tied onto body parts

Purification

In order to purify the supplicant from sins and evil influences, he or she may be sprinkled with blessed and unboiled water on the face, back, under both feet, and on both hands. In the biblical sense the body and in particular the hands or feet may have helped to commit sins and therefore have to be purified. The prophet should bless the water with the following prayer: 'God of Edward Barnabas Lekganyane, I bless this water that everyone who comes here should be healed in the name of Jesus Christ, Amen.'

Emetics and laxatives administered with copious amounts of fluids (often water mixed with salt, oil, vinegar, or ashes), steam baths, and fumigation are procedures by the faith healer and understood by the patient as purifying and cleansing measures to get rid of 'polluting' or otherwise pathogenic substances. Newspapers are cut into strips and blessed so that they can be burned to purify objects and to heal.

Use of Tea, Coffee, or Salt

Coffee and tea with or without milk are used to purify the blood; salt, to clean the stomach and excess bile through vomiting. For example, in the case of an alcoholic, the supplicant drinks once in the morning on the first day of treatment 5 teaspoons of table salt dissolved in a cup of 250 ml cold water. Thereafter he rests for about one hour and when he tries to vomit he drinks 2 teaspoons of Zion black tea. The tea prevents the client from vomiting but will, together with the salt, increase urinating so that the 'poison' in the body (blood) will be removed. Emetics for alcohol abuse include salt, tea and holy lake water; ashes (from burnt offering and herbs) with holy water from a well (and herbs).

Confession

Through confession as a form of ritual vomiting the evil matter in the patient should be eliminated symbolically for real purification. Among Zionists it was stated that confession of sins and faith in God would render the use of the 'medicine' meaningful. Confession alone was believed to heal disease. For example, an alcoholic may confess his problems and sins about his family and drinking alcohol so that God can forgive him. Confession entails speaking out or open admission of anxieties and problems. In the history of the alcoholic, situations of anxiety and depression were followed by alcohol consumption instead of addressing and admitting his or her problems. Being committed to the Zion Christian Church (ZCC) and the regulation not to take alcohol, he experiences without alcohol an accumulating pressure to speak openly about personal relationships to clear his conscience during the day of the confession before the ZCC.

Behavioural Techniques

Confrontation training with forbidden 'food' is, for example, used in the case of cigarette smoking, and aversive conditioning to decrease the reinforcing properties of cannabis. In the case of cannabis the client must eat a teaspoon of strong coffee whenever he wants to smoke. Antabuse for alcohol abuse includes: ashes and herbs secretly poured into alcohol to cause a bad smell and vomiting or beer blessed with holy papers by waving them around it and given to the person to drink. In order to stop someone from smoking the prophet may pray for an unopened packet of cigarettes to produce a bad smell so that the client will refrain from smoking.

Proscriptions

Moral rules among Zionists and Apostolics prohibit smoking, gambling, drinking, and promiscuity, and have a puritan ethic. Members are subject to proscriptions, which usually include an injunction against the consumption of alcoholic beverages and in many cases against the use of other drugs. This religious prohibition is associated with a readiness to rehabilitate a substance-dependent repentant as a patient in the context of the church's healing mandate, usually without charge beyond general tithing (one tenth of the income). A social systems network is established that will provide differential reinforcement contingent upon abstinence and that will facilitate the immediate application of negative consequences contingent upon drinking and/or smoking. Both types of church use a community-reinforcement approach on abstinence from drugs. Additionally, patients take Antabuse and 'lifelong' anti-drug fluids (Peltzer in press).

Indigenous Protective Beliefs such as 'Pollution'

In Malawi, two research sites, one rural (30 km from Zomba) and one urban (Zomba) were chosen to study (in each site) 30 mothers with a malnourished child and 30 control mothers who had no history of malnutrition in their children. According to the mothers in the two sites the concept of the cause of malnutrition was as given in Table 9.2.

Table 9.2   Rural and urban concepts of causes of malnutrition according to their rank

Rural mothers ($n = 60$)	Urban mothers ($n = 60$)
1. Violation of (sexual) rules	1. Lack of food
2. Witchcraft	2. Early or abrupt weaning
3. Natural, God's will	3. Lack of maternal care
4. Lack of food	4. Violation of (sexual) rules

The emic term for malnutrition, *tsempho* and sometimes *mdulo* or *kutumpira*, can be understood by referring to the etiological concept of behavioural (especially sexual) misconduct. Comparing rural or traditional and urban or transitional etiology, it becomes evident that the more traditional the mothers, the more likely they will be to explain malnutrition by violation of sexual rules, and the more modern the mothers, the more likely they will be to refer to 'lack of food' as the primary cause. In particular, extramarital sexual intercourse was seen by many women as a cause of malnutrition.

According to some traditional mothers the child is punished for the mis-behaviour of the mother (and sometimes the father) because the child is considered to be a gift, and if the receiver does not show the necessary appreciation of the child, the gift of the child will be 'removed'. If the mother cooks for the child when she is menstruating, it is believed that her 'hot blood' can cause malnutrition in the child. It is common in all (sexual) rules which are believed to cause malnutrition that the violator gets 'hot blood' when in contact with the child, so causing malnutrition. Where malnutrition was explained as being caused by witchcraft, this usually involves couples who already have several children so that another child resulted in in-creased jealousy of relatives and friends who often do not have children of their own. The concept of 'lack of food', mainly in terms of the three food groups, seems to be a modern concept introduced by modern health services and extension workers.

Little traditional information, which can directly or indirectly be related to nutrition, is given during puberty but it is conveyed mainly during the first pregnancy by elder women, the aunt or grandmother, but not the mother. During the first pregnancy ceremony (*chisamba*) the 8-month expectant woman is advised on the following: not to eat eggs and not to work hard, to take some 'medicine' to protect the fetus from 'witchcraft', and not to have sexual intercourse. Moreover, she is taught how to distinguish different types of crying in the infant, such as crying from hunger, fear, pain or illness. In the case of hunger she should breast-feed on demand. When she is men-struating she is not supposed to cook for the child since her blood is believed to be 'hot'. Finally, she is advised not to have sexual intercourse before the infant is 6–9 months old so as to avoid malnutrition in the child. Almost all rural mothers went through the pregnancy ceremony whereas only 30% of the mothers in town did, and this arose where an aunt came to stay with her or her husband sent her to the village. When the urban woman becomes pregnant without being married, her parents will discard her traditional information. Modern information on nutrition is mainly given at maternity and under-five clinics, agricultural or homecraft extension work, and formal schools, mainly on the three food groups (carbohydrates, proteins, fats), rules of hygiene and breast-feeding (Peltzer 1995).

Another example of an indigenous preventive belief to prevent illicit sex-ual relationships concerns men. Gelfand (1980) describes a belief that pre-vents adultery among the Shona in Zimbabwe. This is if a man develops certain incurable diseases, such as a swollen abdomen, his traditional healer is likely to conclude that he had slept with the wife of an absent husband. The latter, before leaving, must have placed in his bed a special medicine known as *runyoka*. All men know that if they have illicit relations with married women, there is a good chance of their being punished with an illness that is liable to end fatally. The fear of *runyoka* is likely to deter a man who is interested in the wife of another.

THEORETICAL PERSPECTIVES

Green (1997a) states that contagion theory in sub-Saharan Africa comprises at least three types of etiological belief: (1) 'naturalistic infection' or what has been called folk germ theory (e.g. often in the case of sexually transmitted diseases); (2) 'mystical contagion' or pollution; and (3) environmental dangers. The idea behind pollution is that when one comes into physical contact with a substance considered unclean or ritually impure, one becomes sick. Africans believed to be in an unclean or polluted state are often kept apart from others, because they are considered contagious until 'purified', a process that might involve treatment with herbs. For example, in central Mozambique, several kinds of childhood diarrhea are believed to be caused by contact with polluting essences (as well as by eating bad or spoiled food). One source of pollution is unfaithful behaviour on the part of the parent: if a mother or father commits adultery, he or she acquires a contaminating essence that, after physical contact with the child, can make the child sick. This belief tends to reinforce the importance of fidelity in marriage.

A third component of contagion theory, environmental dangers, is based on the belief that elements in the physical environment can cause or spread illness. One expression of the notion is that contagious illness can be carried in the air. For example, the Bemba of Zambia believe that tuberculosis is an 'illness in the air' (*amalwele yamumwela*), spread by inhalation of unclean dust carried by the wind. Colds, influenza, tuberculosis, and some types of contagious childhood diarrhea are examples of illnesses carried by the air and inhaled. Another expression of 'environmental dangers' is based on the notion of balance or adaptation achieved between living beings and their environment. For example, it has been found that when people migrate to or within malarial zones, their lack of resistance to local strains of malaria in the new environment makes them more vulnerable than indigenous people.

Pollution beliefs represent an area of a potential intersectorial interface between indigenous and cosmopolitan medicine. Both are concerned with cleanliness; environmental sanitation; prevention of contact with impurity; contagion and its avoidance; the danger of 'dirt'; and the value of clean, pure food that agrees with the consumer. Both traditional and modern medicine agree that within this domain, the cause of illness is impersonal and relates to conditions that may be modifiable. There seems to be a potential interface in ideas about both contagion and prevention. Therefore, depending on the socio-cultural context public health messages should be framed in terms of appropriate pollution-causality beliefs (Green 1997b).

Jansen (1973) notes that some Xhosa rituals have a protective and preventive significance. For example, young mothers and children wear charms (*ubu-lunga*) around their necks in order to ward off witchcraft influences, as they form an at-risk group to which the activities of witches are directed. *Ubu-lunga* (from *uku-lunga* = to be right) is a necklace made of hair plucked from the tails of cattle. It was an old Xhosa custom to give an *ubu-lunga* animal to the bride who became its personal owner and this cow was held sacred and expressed the close ties between the family and cattle. It is claimed that the wearing of an *ubu-lunga* corrects any evil that may threaten its wearer.

Prevention, in a Western sense, has to do with past–future time orientation, the effect of such medical action being in the remote future, e.g. poliomyelitis vaccination when there is no threat of an epidemic. In an African context the time concept seems to be focused on the present, the cyclical and on a process rather than on an outcome (Peltzer 1995). The traditional African concept of prevention or 'immunization' such as against evil influences of witchcraft is a more situational than a structural matter of countermagic. The Xhosa concept of prevention, for example, is deeply rooted in the belief that the ancestors protect their well-being and that any disorder in tribal life is a sign of a disturbed cosmological balance. Prevention is aimed at propitiating the ancestors, hoping to receive their favours and protection. The Western preventive approach involves more the control of nature and physiological processes. Gelfand (1956: 154) writes in his chapter on preventive medicine: 'The Shona . . . believes that illness caused by magic can be prevented by countermagic and therefore it is essential to protect himself by magical means.'

Van der Geest (1997) believes that most African medical theories have an orientation of prevention. Prevention is central in African people's everyday life and follows logically from their preoccupation with religious and social values. Traditional healers concentrate on the deeper origins of illness and insist that something should be done about them to avoid repetition. They provide their patients with moral and social guidelines to prevent them from catching the same illness.

Another characteristic of African medical theories is that health and illness are more comprehensive concepts than in the Western tradition. In fact, 'health' cannot be adequately translated in many African languages. Indigenous terms closest to it comprise a much wider semantic field. They refer to the general quality of life, including the conditions of animals and plants, the entire physical and social environment. 'Well-being' or even 'happiness' seem better English terms to capture the meaning of traditional African medical concepts. As a consequence, the English term 'medicine' is also a misnomer, but interestingly it has been indigenized in many African languages and now entails much more than restoring bodily health. Medicine is any substance that can bring about a change, anywhere, anyhow. Medicines heal sickness, catch a thief, help someone to pass an exam, make a business prosper, kill an enemy and win someone's love (Van der Geest 1997)). Longmore (1959) has classified various types of African medicines as follows:

- *Assertive medicines*; general, love-philtres, and for professional success. They are supposed to have the effect of making a man popular, liked by everyone, visited by many, listened to by influential neighbours, and successful in all walks of life.
- *Protective medicines* whose function is to protect the consumer, his family, and property, against evil influences.

- *Creative medicines* to produce fertility in men, animals and agriculture.
- *Aggressive medicines* (black magic) for homicide and for bewitching persons or objects.

INSIGHTS, RECOMMENDATIONS AND IMPLICATIONS

Indigenous mechanisms of health promotion in Africa (south of the Sahara) consist of self-care (as it pertains to gender, developmental stages and associated rites of passage, and spirituality, and dreams), mutual aid (as seen in rituals such as in the context of possession cults or social networking) and healthy environments (especially in regard to animals and health and the land and health).

Implementation can be achieved through fostering public participation, strengthening community health services, and coordinating public health policy. This should take several forms as pointed out by the Jakarta Declaration on Health Promotion (1997) and by Jilek (1993):

(1) Universal implementation, at the local level, of a policy of close collaboration between the health system and traditional medicine in general, and between individual health professionals and traditional practitioners in particular.
(2) Consolidation and expansion of partnerships for health between different sectors at all levels of governance and society.
(3) Creation of local operational frameworks for the exchange of health-promoting information.
(4) Increasing community capacity and empowering the individual. Both traditional communication and the new information media support this process. Social, cultural and spiritual resources need to be harnessed in innovative ways.

Westaway *et al.* (1996) studied the expressed health education needs of black adults in urban South Africa. Eighty-six percent of the men and 97% of the women stated that they would like to receive health education. The most frequently mentioned categories were AIDS (32%), specific diseases such as TB (31%), general health, child health, and family planning. There was a lack of interest in nutrition and hygiene education. Respondents tended to choose as preferred health educators a doctor for AIDS, specific diseases and general health, and a nurse for family planning and child health. Although talks and TV/video were the preferred media for delivery, many (21%) preferred the more creative options of dance, song, drama, posters and pictures. Despite radio being the major source of health education coverage, only 0.02% of the respondents expressed interest in this medium.

Green (1985) proposes that health education must begin with (1) an acknowledgement of traditional medical beliefs and practices, (2) the recognition that there is a large number of traditional and faith healers in African communities (generally more than 1:200), (3) encouraging traditional and faith healers to be part of the focus of health education efforts, health education whenever possible building upon rather than directly confronting traditional beliefs and practices. Green (1997a) feels that preventive health education campaigns could adopt the language, metaphors, and symbolism of indigenous contagion theory in order to become more meaningful to the intended audience, and therefore to better motivate adoption of certain behaviours or technologies. Tumwesigye (1996) describes an integrative modern and traditional health-care programme in Uganda to emphasize health education and community-based health care in the prevention of diseases and related problems. The section on health education deals with severe cases of malnutrition, especially in children and pregnant mothers, and communicable diseases—such as sexually transmitted diseases (STDs), diarrhea, vomiting, and worms.

Airhihenbuwa (1995) has applied a conceptual model (the PEN-3 model) to the planning and development of a culturally appropriate health education/promotion programme to child survival intervention in Nigeria. In this context cultural appropriateness of health behaviour was identified by the community (mothers, village health workers, traditional leaders, and local government representatives) after they had been interviewed on positive, existential, and negative health beliefs and practices such as (1) taking fluids during an illness is acceptable, (2) community leaders must be willing and able to take a lead as change agents, (3) giving plantain porridge to children who have diarrhea, (4) the consumption of pap and/or coconut juice during diarrhea, and (5) sexual abstinence during pregnancy (reducing the incidence of pelvic inflammatory disease).

While the above were seen as positive cultural empowerment the following were seen as no threats to health: (1) beads around a child's wrist and/or ankle to ward off evil spirits, (2) post-partum sexual abstinence prevents semen from mixing with breastmilk, and (3) palm oil and indigo serve as a good soothing lotion for measles. Finally, a number of threats to health were identified such as 'immunization may cause disability and/or death in a child', or 'eggs, meat, or chicken cause a baby to be too large to deliver normally'. The recommended intervention was based on whether the beliefs were long-term and historically rooted in tradition and culture or were recent and short-term. Reinforcing or changing long-term cultural beliefs should be addressed through health education in the home (home visits), and/or person-to-person contact in the community. On the other hand, recent and non-traditionally entrenched health beliefs can be addressed through the mass media.

Socio-culturally Informed Health-promotion Interventions

Airhihenbuwa (1989) argues that a conceptual model for health education in African countries must address cultural sensitivity and cultural appropriateness in programme development. The proposed model consits of three dimensions of health beliefs and behavior that are dynamically interrelated and interdependent. These are health education, educational diagnosis of health behaviour and cultural appropriateness of health behavior. Similarly, Ulin (1992) states that AIDS prevention campaigns have not yet taken into account the cultural, social, and economic constraints on most African women's ability to comply with advice to limit partners and use condoms. In the light of the dominant role males have in sexual relations, health-promotion campaigns must focus specifically on addressing at-risk culturally related sexual values and behaviours (Livingston 1992).

Laver, Van der Borne and Kok (1997) describe the utilization of social change theory and an ecological model for health promotion to develop a participatory intervention for HIV/AIDS prevention in farm workers in Zimbabwe. This involves the need to focus attention on the process of change at the interpersonal, organizational and policy levels of the community. Dialogue is central to the range of strategies proposed for this intervention. Kawewe (1996) proposes a social-networking approach to combat HIV/AIDS in Zimbabwe that is culturally friendly and sensitive to Zimbabwean families. It is suggested that this approach will strengthen the currently isolated traditional family systems by informally connecting extended families with a large national community.

In South Africa, Toroyan and Reddy (1997/1998) found on the basis of a photocomic AIDS intervention that identification with the comic was stronger among Coloured and African youth than that among their White counterparts, supporting the theory that involving the target group in developing health messages will result in a product that is most effective among that particular readership.

Janz *et al.* (1996) evaluated 37 AIDS prevention projects and identified the following socio-cultural factors that facilitated intervention effectiveness identified by staff in the United States: (1) design culturally relevant and appropriate language, (2) embed AIDS information into broader contexts, (3) provide creative rewards and enticements, (4) build in opportunities for program flexibility, (5) promote integration into and acceptance by the community, (6) repeat essential AIDS prevention messages, (7) create a forum for open discussion, and (8) solicit participant involvement. For example, designing culturally relevant and language-appropriate interventions may include paying attention to the norms, values and traditions of the target population, combining vernacular with formal terminology in important terms and concepts, and soliciting input and participation from the members of the target population.

As an example, the South African government produced a manual on all HIV/AIDS-related terms in all eleven official languages. These facilitating factors should be considered when designing and evaluating health-promotion intervention programs in African socio-cultural contexts. Attitudes of participants towards the intervention activity may differ and have to be considered. For example, MacLachlan (1997) reported that Malawian secondary school pupils repeatedly enjoyed the educational 'AIDS Challenge' board game which they developed, and Bosompra (1991/1992) found among Ghanaian communities that they preferred drama to songs as media for AIDS messages.

EVALUATION OF INTERVENTION ACTIVITIES

Few health-promotion intervention projects have been undertaken in Africa considering the extent of the problem and compared to industrial countries like the United States. The different intervention activities reported for Africa include more commonly awareness campaigns, the distribution of educational materials, the development of new educational materials such as photocomics or board games, drama and theatre, training of peers, condom promotion, and, less commonly, training of professionals including traditional healers, HIV testing, small-group discussions and individual counselling. Most intervention activities perceived to be the most effective in African samples have also been found in other studies to result in knowledge, attitude, and behavior change (Janz et al. 1996). Drama, theatre, photocomics and multifaceted intervention activities have been reported as particularly effective in African contexts (Bosompra 1991/1992, Dalrymple and Du Toit 1993; Klepp et al. 1997; Toroyan and Reddy 1997/1998). Learning theory suggests that people are more likely to learn when messages are presented in multiple formats using different communication strategies (Clark 1987).

CONCLUSION

Sillitoe (1998) argues for the development of indigenous knowledge as a new applied anthropology. It is increasingly acknowledged beyond anthropology that other people have their own effective 'science' and resource-use practices and that to assist them we need to understand something about their knowledge and management systems. The notion of technology transfer remains not as a top-down imposition but as a search for jointly negotiated advances. Participatory approaches seek a more systematic accommodation of indigenous knowledge in research on health interventions. The process of engaging the teachers/interventionists and the students/ audiences in the production of meaning, value, pleasure, and knowledge should be central to the mission of health education. It is only through such a dialogue where varied cultural expressions are affirmed and centralized that the production of a cultural identity can be legitimating and empowering relative to health promotion. This empowerment model of health education intervention focuses on facilitating individual and community choices by supplementing knowledge acquisition with value clarification and decision-making practice and community-organizing skills through non-traditional teaching methods (Airhihenbuwa 1994).

Thus, it is hoped that the rich indigenous mechanisms of promoting health in Africa are empowered and utilized.

REFERENCES

Airhihenbuwa, C.O. (1989) Perspectives on AIDS in Africa: strategies for prevention and control. *AIDS Education and Prevention*, 1, 57–69.

Airhihenbuwa, C.O. (1993) Health promotion for child survival in Africa: implications for cultural appropriateness. *Hygie*, 12, 10–15.

Airhihenbuwa, C.O. (1994) Health promotion and the discourse on culture: implications for empowerment. *Health Education Quarterly*, 21, 345–353.

Banks, W.J. (1998) Emancipatory potential of storytelling in a group. *Journal of Nursing Science* 30, 17–21.

Bosompra, K. (1991/92) The potential of drama and songs as channels for AIDS education in Africa: a report on focus group findings from Ghana. *International Quarterly of Community Health Education*, 12, 317–342.

Bührmann, M.V. (1984) *Living in Two Worlds: Communication between a white healer and her black counterparts.* Cape Town: Human & Rousseau.

Clark, N.M. (1987) Social learning theory in current health education practice. *Advances in Health Education and Promotion*, 2, 251–275.

Dalrymple, L. and Du Toit, M.K. (1993) The evaluation of a drama approach to AIDS education. *Educational Psychology* 13, 147–154.

Gelfand, M. (1956) *Medicine and Magic of the Mashona.* Johannesburg: Juta.

Gelfand, M. (1980) African customs in relation to preventive medicine. *The Central African Journal of Medicine* 27, 1–9.

Green, E.C. (1985) Traditional healers, mothers and childhood diarrheal disease in Swaziland: the interface of anthropology and health education. *Social Science & Medicine*, 20, 277–285.

Green, E.C. (1997a) Is there a basis for modern-traditional cooperation in African health promotion. *The Journal of Alternative and Complementary Medicine*, 3, 311–314.

Green, E.C. (1997b) Purity, pollution and the invisible snake in Southern Africa. *Medical Anthropology*, 17, 83–100.

Jakarta Declaration on Leading Health Promotion (1997) The Jakarta Declaration on Leading Health Promotion into the 21st Century. *Health Promotion International*, 12, 261–264.

Jansen, G. (1973) *The Doctor–patient Relationship in an African Tribal Society.* Assen.

Janz, N.K., Zimmerman, M.A., Israel, B.A., Freudenberg, N. and Carter, R.J. (1996) Evaluation of 37 AIDS prevention projects: successful approaches and barriers to program effectiveness. *Health Education Quarterly*, 23, 80–97.

Jilek, W.G. (1993) Traditional medicine relevant to psychiatry. In N. Sartorius *et al.* (Eds) *Treatment of Mental Disorders* (pp. 341–390). Geneva: WHO/Washington: American Psychiatric Press.

Katz, R. and Wexler, A. (1989) Healing and transformation: lessons from indigenous people (Botswana). In K. Peltzer and P.O. Ebigbo (Eds) *Clinical Psychology in Africa* (pp. 19–43). Frankfurt/M: IKO Verlag.

Kawewe, S.M. (1996) Social-networking Zimbabwean families: an African traditional approach to waging a war against HIV/AIDS. *Social Development Issues*, 18, 34–51.

Klepp, K.-I., Ndeki, S.S., Leshbari, M.T., Hannan, P.J. and Lyimo, B.A. (1997) AIDS education in Tanzania: promoting risk reduction among primary school children. *American Journal of Public Health*, 87, 1931–1936.

Laver, S.M.L., Van der Borne, B. and Kok, G. (1995) Using theory to design an intervention for HIV/AIDS prevention in farm workers in rural Zimbabwe. *International Quarterly of Community Health Education*, 15, 349–362.

Livingston, I.L. (1993) HIV/AIDS control in Africa: the importance of epidemiological and health promotion approaches. *Health Promotion International*, 8, 189–198.

Longmore, L. (1959) *The Dispossessed*. London: Transworld Publishers.

MacLachlan, M. (1997) *Culture and Health*. Chichester: Wiley.

MacLachlan, M., Chimombo, M. and Mpemba, N. (1997) AIDS education for youth through active learning: a school-based approach from Malawi. *International Journal of Educational Development*, 17, 41–50.

Obisesan, K.A., Adeyemo, A.A., Ohaeri, J.U., Aramide, F.A. and Okafor, S.I. (1997) The family planning aspects of the practice of traditional healers in Ibadan, Nigeria. *West African Journal of Medicine*, 16, 184–190.

Peltzer, K. (1987) *Traditional Healing and Psychosocial Health Care in Malawi*. Heidelberg: Asanger.

Peltzer, K. (1990) Dreams, stories and proverbs in a Yoruba village (Nigeria): a psychohygienic perspective. *Sociologus*, 40, 179–190.

Peltzer, K. (1995) *Psychology and Health in African Cultures*. Frankfurt/M: IKO Verlag.

Peltzer, K. (1996) *Counselling and Psychotherapy of Victims of Organised Violence in Sociocultural Context*. Frankfurt/M: IKO Verlag.

Peltzer, K. (in press) Faith healing for mental and social disorders in the Northern Province (South Africa). *Journal of Religion in Africa*.

Pickering, H., Quigley, M., Pepin, J., Todd, J. *et al.* (1993) The effects of post-test counselling on condom use among prostitutes in The Gambia. *AIDS*, 7, 271–273.

Sillitoe, P. (1998) The development of indigenous knowledge. *Current Anthropology*, 39, 223–235.

Toroyan, T. and Reddy, P.S. (1997/98) Participation of South African youth in the design and development of AIDS photocomics. *International Quarterly of Community Health Education*, 17, 131–146.

Tsala Tsala, J. (1998) In S.N. Madu, P.K. Baguma and A. Pritz (eds) *In Quest for Psychotherapy for Modern Africa* (Proceedings of the first conference on psychotherapy in Kampala 1997), Sovenga, South Africa: University of the North.

Tumwesigye, O. (1996) Bumetha Rukararwe: integrating modern and traditional health care in Southwest Uganda. *Journal of Alternative and Complementary Medicine*, 2, 373–376.

Ulin, P.R. (1992) African women and AIDS: negotiating behavioural change. *Social Science & Medicine*, 34, 63–73.

Van der Geest, S. (1997) Is there a role for traditional medicine in basic health services in Africa? A plea for a community perspective. *Tropical Medicine & International Health*, 2, 903–911.

Westaway, M.S., Wolmarans, L., Wessie, G.M. and Viljoen, E. (1996) Expressed health education needs of black adults living in Ivory Park (Gauteng). *Curationis*, 19, 71–73.

Chapter 10

Cultivating the Psychosocial Health of Refugees

Alastair Ager and Marta Young

CASE STUDY*

Francine Mukandori is a 27-year-old Rwandan woman who is claiming refugee status in Canada. She was referred to a psychologist by her immigration lawyer for a psychological evaluation. During the first interview session, Mrs Mukandori was distressed and tearful as she told her story. She was born in Uganda to Rwandan parents where she lived with her family as *de facto* refugees until the age of 13. Her parents belonged to the Tutsi tribe and were forced to flee Rwanda in the 1950s due to rising ethnic tensions between the Tutsis and the Hutus. In 1982, Mrs Mukandori's family, along with other Rwandan refugees, were repatriated to Rwanda. While she described life during her teenage and young adult years in Rwanda as relatively peaceful, she did report widespread discrimination on the part of Hutus towards Tutsis. In 1989, at the age of 20, Mrs Mukandori married and had two children, a daughter and a son. Into the 1990s, Mrs Mukandori reported an increase in tension between the Tutsis and the Hutus and the beginning of a general climate of violence. Her parents were forced to move villages for their own protection and Mrs Mukandori and her family went to live with them.

April 1994 heralded the start of horrific genocidal massacres in various villages, including the one where Mrs Mukandori and her family were staying. Early one morning, all the Tutsi and Tutsi-friendly villagers were rounded up in

---

* This case study is an anonomised account of clinical experience of the second author. An elaboration of this case study—and its subsequent analysis is provided in Loughry and Ager (1999).

Cultivating Health: Cultural Perspectives on Promoting Health. Edited by M. MacLachlan.
© 2001 John Wiley & Sons Ltd.

the village square by Hutu militiamen and were asked to form two lines. Mrs Mukandori, her husband and two children along with several siblings were put in one line, the rest of her family, including her mother, father, and brother were placed in the other line, and the slaughter of the villagers began. Mrs Mukandori and her immediate family, including her two small children, witnessed the dismemberment and killing with machetes of her mother, father and brother. Another brother and two sisters were also killed that morning but Mrs Mukandori did not witness their deaths. Towards the end of the massacre, a youth involved in the killing approached Mrs Mukandori and identified himself as a friend of the family. He rounded up Mrs Mukandori, her husband and, children as well as three remaining sisters aged 10 to 18. He told his Hutu friends that he was planning to kill them and there was no need for them to wait for him. As a sign of his intent to follow through with the killings, he told Mrs Mukandori's husband that he was planning to cut him piece by piece and then proceeded to cut off one of his fingers in front of his friends. When his friends finally departed, he helped Mrs Mukandori's remaining family to escape to safety.

They lived in an attic-like space of an old abandoned house where they remained with little water, milk or food. After approximately ten days, the level of tension and stress, not to mention the lack of food and water, was such that the children were having great difficulty in coping with the situation. Mrs Mukandori and her husband decided to risk coming out. As they wandered the countryside, they realized that the massacres had continued while they had been in hiding. Fresh mutilated bodies were strewn throughout the area, including the one of the Hutu youth who had spared their lives. Mrs Mukandori and her family continued to fear for their lives and eventually decided to relocate to another part of Rwanda where they lived for the following three years.

While they lived in relative peace during those years, incidents of Tutsis 'disappearing' or being killed were common. In 1997, several unknown armed men knocked at their door and asked to speak with her husband. He was ordered into a car and whisked away. Two days later, the same men came back to Mrs Mukandori's home and told her that they had killed her husband and that if she told anyone she would be next. Mrs Mukandori was very frightened and she decided it was time to flee. Along with her two young children and youngest sister, she travelled over 300 kilometres on foot and with the help of various modes of transportation including minibuses and motorcycles. Their escape route eventually took them to a Rwanda–Zaire bordertown where they arrived late one evening. As it was too late to cross the border, she approached an elderly man and his wife and asked them if they would be willing to put them up for the night, a request to which they willingly agreed. After spending the evening sharing with her hosts the various events that had brought her to flee, Mrs Mukandori decided to leave her children and sister in the care of this couple, as the border crossing was fraught with danger. Her plan was to have them join her once she had reached a safe haven. After a harrowing trek during which she was shot at and nearly raped by armed bandits, she finally made her way to the Zairean capital. After a few days, she was able to trace some distant relatives who helped her to cover the costs of an air ticket and a fake Dutch passport. After an agonizing week dealing with the separation from her children as well as with the multiple preparations required to flee Zaire, she boarded a plane for Canada and arrived in May 1997 claiming refugee status.

With respect to her current emotional state, Mrs Mukandori described often telling herself that she has to forget the past. In the same breath, however, she admitted to not being able to do so in that she has recurring intrusive thoughts about the massacre of her parents and siblings, the death of her husband, and the separation from her children. Mrs Mukandori described feelings of sadness and being very worried about her children's safety in Rwanda. 'I have nothing left now, not even my family.' She also described significant problems in that her mind often wanders back to the traumatic events she experienced in Rwanda. 'When this happens, I push these memories away and force myself to concentrate.' Mrs Mukandori also presented with chronic sleep difficulties in that she cannot fall asleep before midnight and then awakens 3 or 4 hours later, unable to fall asleep again. She described being so afraid at night that she has to keep all the lights on. She also has frequent nightmares in which she sees men coming to get her husband or she relives the slaughter of her family and neighbours. She typically wakes up from these nightmares shaking and in terror. Other residents of the shelter where she is currently staying have reported how they hear her scream in her sleep.

In addition to these psychological difficulties, Mrs Mukandori is also confronted with a number of significant acculturative and psychosocial stressors. While she is grateful for the safety that living in Canada brings to her, Mrs Mukandori experiences great difficulty in adjusting to a new culture and climate. She only speaks a few words of English and no French, finds the winters cold and isolating, and has been the victim of discrimination (e.g. racial slurs, being rudely spoken to by a bus conductor, being ignored in a grocery store). Furthermore, Mrs Mukandori finds Canadian norms, values, and customs strange and unfamiliar, and government agencies confusing. In particular, she often finds herself in situations where she has difficulty in deciphering Canadians' non-verbal behaviour, where she is unclear about gender and family roles, and where she has difficulty in knowing which social service agency to contact due to uncertainty regarding their various mandates. Financially, she has no sources of income, except for a small allowance from the Government. Consequently, she lives in an overcrowded shelter for homeless women, and relies on foodbanks and other community resources to feed and clothe herself.

This 27-year-old Rwandan woman is a survivor of war trauma (witnessing killings, dead bodies, stresses related to fleeing), and has experienced multiple concomitant losses (of parents, siblings, husband, homeland and separation from her children). While the utility of such a diagnosis can be contested, her current emotional status meets all the criteria for Post-Traumatic Stress Disorder of chronic duration (i.e. more than 3 months) with depressed mood as outlined in the Diagnostic and Statistical Manual of Mental Disorders (DSM-IV). In particular, the war trauma witnessed is re-experienced by recurrent and intrusive nightmares and distress when exposed to stimuli that remind her of

the war. She also exhibits symptoms of increased arousal, such as sleep difficulties, hypervigilance and difficulty in concentrating. As is common in sur-
vivors of extensive trauma, Mrs Mukandori's main coping strategy is to
emotionally numb the pain experienced by isolating her affect by avoiding
thinking about the trauma, and by having complete or partial amnesia about
the incidents. These coping strategies are effective in containing the intense
feelings and help her to maintain a semblance of normality in her daily life,
though they constrain her capacity to meaningfully engage in her new
environment.

Upon completion of psychological assessment, it was recommended that
Mrs Mukandori be accepted as a bona fide refugee. In due course, and in
recognition of other relevant appraisals, the Immigration and Refugee Board
granted her refugee status in Canada in 1998. While she no longer lives with
the precarious status of being a refugee claimant, she continues to experience
severe emotional and behavioural symptoms, she is still separated from her
children and remaining family back in central Africa, and she faces the challenges of adjusting culturally, linguistically and economically to Canada.

THE DIMENSIONS OF THE REFUGEE EXPERIENCE

The experience of Mrs Mukandori is clearly unique in its detail and yet it
vividly illustrates the range of challenges to psychosocial well-being commonly faced by forced migrants. Mrs Mukandori is one of some 50 million
persons who are currently displaced from their homes internally within a
nation-state or across international borders as a result of military conflict,
political persecution or ethnic violence (Westin 1999). Some half of these, by
crossing international borders in search of protection, fall within the terms of
the 1951 Geneva Convention and thus within the formal remit of the United
Nations High Commissioner for Refugees or UNHCR (Zetter 1999). The
legal status of the remainder—displaced within the borders of their own
country—is less clear, through their vulnerabilities in psychosocial terms
may be considered similar.

While a number of features within Mrs Mukandori's experience will be
shown to be recurrent, one key feature of her story is statistically atypical.
Refugees reaching countries of the industrialised world and seeking asylum
remain—notwithstanding media representations to the contrary (Westin
1999)—significantly in the minority. The vast majority of forced migrants
who do flee across an international border do so to a neighbouring country,
and from this neighbouring country the most frequent 'durable solution' to
their displacement is subsequent repatriation back to their home nation.

In such circumstances it may be tempting to distinguish between analysis
of the 'Western-resettling' refugee and the forced migrant enduring temporary settlement in a neighbouring country before returning—at the end of
the prevailing conflict—to their homeland. Such a distinction would, for
example, usefully highlight the influence of such factors as 'cultural

distance' (the difference between home- and host-cultures) on refugee adjustment. Clearly the challenges faced by Mrs Mukandori in Canada now are quite distinct from those faced by her surviving relatives in Rwanda.

Yet analysis of the experience of refugees across a broad range of settings (Ager 1999; Marsella *et al.* 1994) suggests sufficient commonality in the issues addressed in such adaptation and adjustment—if not the circumstances themselves—to make a single framework of analysis appropriate. Issues of fear, identity and belonging are played out in an infinite variety of cultural contexts and yet remain key challenges for the majority of forced migrants. In such circumstances, it makes sense to avoid any over-simplified division of refugee experience—and mechanisms supporting refugees' psychosocial health—into that of the 'developed' and 'developing' worlds, but rather seek a holistic analysis of factors impacting adjustment, reflecting the unique cultural contexts and demands faced by each displaced person.

From the perspective of considering the discrete psychological and social challenges faced by refugees, four discrete phases of the refugee experience may usefully be distinguished (Ager 1999). The *pre-flight* phase refers to the period leading up to flight itself. This may be an extended period and may feature economic hardship, social disruption, physical violence and political oppression. This phase may bring extreme physical suffering (e.g. torture) and considerable anguish regarding the decision to flee one's home, possessions, land etc. Three years separated the death the of Mrs Mukandori's parents and her final decision to flee across the border to Zaire. Mozambican refugees reported months of living in the mountains above their home village, hiding from military forces, before their ultimate decision to leave their homeland for neighbouring Malawi (Ager, Ager and Long 1995). Doná and Berry (1999) report the economic and social deprivation of Guatemalan tribal peoples who faced the oppression of a hostile government rather than abandon their land in following others to refuge in Mexico.

The subsequent *flight* phase then involves the experience of separation from home (and frequently family), and the dangers of passage itself to a country of first asylum. Many refugees face extremely hazardous journeys during flight. The flight of the Vietnamese boat people represents one of the most arduous journeys in seeking refuge (Ager 1999). Mrs Mukandori's 300-kilometre flight by foot and motor vehicle, followed by the hazards of the border crossing, may be considered a somewhat more typical journey, though many women report the occurrence rather than the threat of sexual assault in securing a safe passage (Callamard 1999).

The phase which follows flight—that of *temporary settlement or asylum-seeking*—may involve extended accommodation in a formal refugee camp or centre, where the routines of normal life are hard to establish. While safe from the threats that characterised life in the home country, the processes of negotiating assistance, legal recognition, family reunification etc. in the country of asylum are frequently experienced as highly stressful, with the conditions and circumstances of many refugee camps significantly adding to this. Many asylum-seekers experience the 'limbo' of this phase for many years, uncertain of their long-term future and the likelihood of being forced

to return to their home country. For Mrs Mukandori the process of ad-
judicating on her asylum application took in the order of one year. In many
countries the process is considerably longer than this. Even in (the majority
of) settings where refugees seek not formal asylum status, but leave to
remain in safety from a neighbouring conflict, uncertainty and ambiguity
about the future can be a major issue. Refugees frequently report the fear of
forcible repatriation to their home country, a fear which has sometimes been
fueled by the actions of host governments and agencies (Westin 1999).

The final phase of the refugee experience involves *resettlement* or *repatriation*. As noted earlier, increasingly few asylum-seekers are now accepted as
formal refugees with rights to permanently resettle within a country of
asylum. Repatriation to the country of origin is increasingly seen by governments as the most appropriate 'durable solution' to forced migration movements. Evidence (Majodina 1999; Doná and Berry 1999) suggests that on
repatriation refugees frequently experience considerable difficulties in re-
entry and re-adjustment with, in some circumstances, the threats which
encouraged flight potentially remaining. Resettlement itself, however, commonly brings such challenges as racism, employment difficulties (with frequent downward mobility within the employment market) and culture
conflicts (particularly inter-generational stresses with the differential socialisation of parents and children within the host society). Such issues are
clear or implicit in much of Mrs Mukandori's experience in Canada. The
challenge is not just to her current state of well-being. The disjuncture between her own cultural values and socialisation history, and that of the
culture around her, threatens her longer-term identity and her capacity to
act coherently and meaningfully in this setting.

THE GROWTH OF PSYCHOSOCIAL PROGRAMMING

The potential impact on the well-being of refugees of the range of challenges
outlined above has been appreciated for many years. Conceptualising such
impact in particularly psychosocial terms dates from at least the 1930s. A
study published in 1939 regarding the adjustment in the United States of
refugees from Nazi Germany notes:

> 'some of the everyday ways of living that are new and confusing; indicates
> some of the more fundamental questions he [sic] faces; and suggests the psy-
> chosocial sources of such characteristics as over-aggressiveness.' (Kraus 1939)

Psychosocial analysis—although often used as a term in different ways by
differing workers—generally refers to experience that is particularly influenced by the interaction of the psychological and social worlds of an individual. Mrs Mukandori's psychological state subsequent to her bereavement,
separation and cultural isolation clearly interacts with her capacity to deal
effectively with her social world. Equally, the social demands made upon her
(and, crucially, the social supports she receives) will impact her psychological

well-being. It is the interplay of such social and psychological forces which determines the status of a person's psychosocial well-being.

Approaches to supporting the psychosocial well being of forced migrants accordingly reflect emphasis on both social and more personal, psychological factors. While there is sometimes considered a tension between social and more psychological approaches (Summerfield 1999; Ager 1997), it is likely that approaches which acknowledge the interaction of social and personal worlds are the most effective. Nor would the separation of programming into rigid categories of 'social' or 'psychological' be that straightforward. Many psychosocial programmes in Croatia and Bosnia-Herzegovina, which have been described in broadly psychological terms, in practice incorporated a good deal of community development activity, including the formation of income-generating cooperatives (Agger 1995). In programmes which did feature explicit counseling or psychotherapy sessions, beneficiaries commonly rated such activities as of lesser significance than group work or community-focused activity (Agger and Mimeca 1996).

While it is argued here that psychosocial intervention appropriately integrates social and psychological approaches to the prevention of mental health problems and social difficulties, it is appropriate to note the increased 'psychologisation' of the discourse regarding such work over the last sixty years. In fact, conceptual development in the field of psychosocial intervention in this period has been marked by two phenomena. One is this increased emphasis by agencies and assistance workers on more psychological accounts in appraising the well-being of forced migrants; the other is the shift in the conceptualisation of refugees by agencies, policy makers and researchers towards analysis of refugee communities and populations, rather than individual refugees. Thus at the beginning of this period the account of refugee adjustment provided by Kraus presents psychosocial well-being as very much reflecting successful assimilation of the individual refugee into the new host culture, urging persons to:

'see him [sic], not at the end of a road, defeated, but at the beginning of his American career, a budding American citizen, eager to assume and share all the responsibilities of a new homeland.' (Kraus 1939).

Many assumptions and constructions within this quotation conflict with current views and expectations of refugees held by agencies, assistance workers and, indeed, refugees themselves. There is little attention paid in this quotation to the broader social links of the refugee within their own community of origin. The circumstances of the refugee are considered in very much individual (male) terms while conceptualisation of their needs is very much focused on issues of employment and accommodation. There is little attention paid to the 'inner experience' of the refugee.

The focus on individual—rather than community- or population-level—adjustment continued in work examining the psychosocial consequences of forced displacement following the Second World War. The Geneva Convention on Refugees of 1951 had, indeed, served to enshrine the rights of individuals with a 'well found fear of persecution'. The work of authors such as Murphy (1955) and Krupinski, Stoller and Wallace (1973) remained focused on outcomes for individual refugees resettling in host countries. There was some sign of the 'psychologisation' of refugee needs in such work, though this tended to be within the structure of established psychiatric diagnoses such as depression and schizophrenia. Such work demonstrated the long-term vulnerability of refugees to mental health problems, in comparison to the population within which they had resettled.

Through the course of the 1970s research studies—and the intervention programmes then frequently related to—began to demonstrate a different character. Refugee movements from, for instance, South-East Asia resulted in the displacement of significant numbers of the Vietnamese, Hmong, Laotian and Kmer communities of that region. Such movements increasingly strained the definitions and procedures for granting asylum and resettlement established in the immediate post-Second World War context (Zetter 1999). Refugees in such contexts were increasingly acknowledged as representing migrant 'communities' with distinctive needs—and resources—of their own; rather than an agglomeration of individuals to be assimilated into host societies. Assistance programmes for such refugees began to take on a character more associated with current psychosocial approaches. Emphasis on community development and the establishment of mutual assistance agencies (MAAs) grew (McCallin 1996).

As suggested previously, this evolution of approach was marked not only by a greater appreciation of the community context of refugees but also by an increasing tendency to address psychological aspects of refugee adjustment. The work of Kinzie (Kinzie *et al.* 1990; Kinzie and Sack 1991) and Mollica (Mollica et al. 1987; Mollica, Wyshak and Lavelle 1993) was particularly influential in suggesting that the experience of many refugees may be appropriately conceptualised within the emerging framework of post-traumatic stress disorder (PTSD). Kinzie, for example, established that 50% of Cambodian children attending schools in Oregon met the diagnostic criteria for PTSD. Such findings fostered not only a greater emphasis on psychological functioning of refugees, it also established interest in 'outreach' and health-promotion programmes, seeking to support the social well-being of refugees who were not necessarily presenting to health and social welfare services.

This interest in conceptualisations such as PTSD has continued to the present day, but psychosocial work with refugees has—since the mid-1980s—had to adjust to the global trend noted at the beginning of this chapter. While the number of refugees has grown steadily through this period, the proportion that are involved in resettlement in a third country within the developed world has decreased appreciably. Thus the key psychosocial challenge globally is not addressing the needs of refugees resettling from the developing world (or, indeed, from transitional economies in Eastern Europe) to the developed world. Rather, it is the support of refugees displaced within a region, with the people involved in such population movements now typically (e.g. Afghanistan, Rwanda, Kosovo etc.) numbered in hundreds of thousands. (This is not to say that such 'within-region' displacement is a new phenomenon. Rather such movements have become—very much for political reasons (Westin 1999)—the focus of attention for international agencies and researchers, previously generally inattentive to forced migration within the developing world.)

Refugee movements need now to be understood in terms not only of communities (which remains important) but also of major populations. Such a trend has put further strain on the Geneva Convention as a base for legal recognition of refugees, and not only because of its phrasing in terms of 'an individual . . . with a well-found fear of persecution'. Persons displaced *within the borders* of their own country (typically referred to as 'internally displaced persons') are not formally recognised as refugees by the convention, but face—from a psychosocial, and often political, perspective—very similar challenges to those who have formally crossed international borders.

Psychosocial programming in this context has generally had to adopt 'population-level' interventions, whether this involves strengthening community structures and activities or intervening through the support and training of teachers or other personnel (Richman 1993; Ager 1997). Attempts at addressing the individual, psychological needs of refugees are clearly challenged by the scale of such population movements. However, many psychosocial programmes have constructed their interventions with respect to variations on the 'pyramidal' structure of population need and response (Mollica 1994; Adjukovic and Adjukovic 1998). This suggests that population-level interventions address the needs of the majority of refugees, but that appropriate assessment and referral mechanisms are put in place to provide more specialised services to the minority of people who require such additional support. Many interventions—particularly in emergency circumstances—now involve some appreciation of such a 'bi-phasic' or phased response to psychosocial needs (Ager 1995, 1997).

The last sixty years has thus seen a development in our understanding of the psychosocial needs of refugees, and in responses to such needs. Reflecting trends in forced migration in the latter half of the twentieth century, refugee movements have increasingly been understood in terms of displaced populations rather than individual refugees. Refugees' experience has, in the same period, increasingly been considered in psychological as well as broader social terms. While these general trends are apparent, there continues to be a wide range of theoretical perspectives influencing contemporary psychosocial programming. Closer analysis of such perspectives is considered in the next section

CURRENT THEORETICAL PERSPECTIVES

Psychiatry

Psychiatry continues to have a significant influence on the appraisal of psychosocial need and conceptualisation of appropriate means of addressing such need. It was noted earlier how work such as that of Murphy (1955) used diagnostic criteria for psychoses such as depression and schizophrenia as a means of appraising refugee adjustment on resettlement. Such diagnostic categories are now rarely given prominence in appraisal of the mental health status of refugees. Post-traumatic stress disorder (PTSD) has become the most frequently screened-for psychiatric diagnosis (Van der Veer 1998), as well as a concept utilised in the planning of many intervention programmes (Agger 1995; Joseph, Williams and Yule 1999).

It was noted earlier that Mrs Mukandori meets all the criteria for a diagnosis of PTSD as defined by the fourth revision of the Diagnostic and Statistical Manual of Mental Disorders of the American Psychiatric Association (DSM-IV). This diagnostic category, however, was originally conceived (and is still more generally used) to describe a pattern of symptoms arising from a single traumatic event. Many refugees, as with Mrs Mukandori, have in fact faced a whole series of events which would generally be perceived to be traumatic in nature, with many current stressors adding to their difficulties of emotional adjustment. Some adopting a psychiatric formula to appraise the psychosocial needs of refugees are thus coming to favour alternative diagnostic categories available within the WHO's International Classification of Disease (ICD) to represent more accurately the experience of refugees.

As will be noted later, the use of any form of psychiatric classification to appraise refugees' needs has been widely critiqued. Such categorisation risks decontextualising suffering, devaluing personal understandings, and de-emphasising the material and social factors that would appropriately be addressed to mitigate suffering (Muecke 1992; Bracken, Giller and Summerfield 1995). However, the use of such classification remains widespread. It is somewhat remarkable that this remains the case when such categorisation does so little to inform the precise strategy or method of intervention. Generally very few psychosocial programmes adopt a classic psychiatric approach to treatment, either through pharmacology or psychotherapy. It appears that psychiatric classification is predominantly used as a means of quantifying need (often in broad public health terms) rather than directing treatment.

Counselling

This is not to say that psychotherapeutic intervention is not articulated as a potential response to the psychosocial needs of refugees. Counselling has been suggested as a key provision by many arguing that such intervention can support adjustment (Agger 1997; Van der Veer 1998). Other than in a very small minority of situations where refugees are consulting therapists in specialised units for, for example, the victims of torture, the counselling provided within psychosocial programmes does not involve an intensive psychotherapeutic intervention clearly predicated upon a established psychiatric diagnosis. Counselling is generally promoted as a more generalised supportive intervention, encouraging refugees to articulate aspects of their experience and identify developmental goals for themselves. There are many examples of such counselling interventions with regard to interventions in Croatia and Bosnia-Herzegovina (Agger 1995; Adjukovic and Adjukovic 1998). Such interventions include group counselling, particularly that seeking to facilitate the empowerment of participants. Where such interventions occur, it may be difficult to discern the bass of their potential effectiveness. Data cited by Agger and Mimeca (1996) suggests, for example, that participants rated the opportunity to share together with others their experience more useful than counselling and therapeutic work (though it is unclear how facilitative of group sharing the counselling may itself have been).

Social Psychology

Social psychology has influenced the conceptualisation of support for forced migrants adjusting to a new environment, principally through the work of John Berry (Berry 1992; Doná and Berry 1999). It was noted previously that Mrs Mukandori faces a range of challenges in acculturating within the host environment of Canada. Berry has proposed that the process—and, ultimately, the outcomes—of acculturation of migrant groups within a host culture is principally determined by two factors. One is the degree of contact the group has with the host culture; the other is the value that is placed on the group retaining its discrete cultural identity. Where a group has close contact with a host culture, and there is concern to retain pre-existing cultural identity, the pattern conforms to the acculturative process of *assimilation*. Where there is minimal contact with the host culture, and concern to retain pre-existing identity, the pattern is one of *separation*. Such processes are often seen as determined by the aspirations of the migrant group, but clearly the pattern followed is also heavily influenced by the expectations of the host community.

Berry's framework has had a significant influence on research work in the area. It has also, however, been used as a framework to plan interventions which support what is considered by Berry to be the most satisfactory acculturative pattern for the psychosocial well-being of migrant groups—that of *integration*. This represents the pattern where a migrant group seeks (or is encouraged towards) frequent contact with the host culture, but retains value in its pre-existing values and identity. Given the evidence that cultural contact can challenge and distort value systems and cultural practices of a minority group (Doná and Berry 1999), this goal involves fostering structures, rituals and rhythms which protect social identity within an 'alien' environment. Activities targeted at protecting social, cultural, and religious practice among youths within displaced communities (Ressler, Boothby and Steinbock 1988) may be seen to be particularly supporting an integrational form of acculturation.

Although the acculturation literature may be considered to be particularly relevant in the case of refugees resettling long-term in host countries, the analysis is also helpful in suggesting appropriate policy and practice in countries of temporary asylum. Even short periods within a dominant host culture may be seen to undermine the cultural identity of a migrant group unless care is taken to preserve key routines and practices within the temporary environment. Where host governments seek to minimise 'cross-contamination' of cultures by minimising contact between groups, identity may be preserved, but at the cost of significant social, economic and political deprivation.

Developmental Psychology

Children have been perceived as a particularly vulnerable group within displaced communities, and have thus been a particular focus for psychosocial intervention in many settings (Ahearn, Loughry and Agar 1999; McCallin 1996). Principles of developmental psychology have been a major influence on the goals and methods of such interventions. Displacement is seen as a threat to the social, emotional and intellectual development of children because of the disruption of the environment in which the child is socialised (Ager 1995). Interventions are therefore commonly framed in terms of the restoration of an environment in which the child can resume developmental progress. This obviously includes the support—where attainable—of family reunification and, more generally, the rebuilding of communities. In addition, however, programmes may seek more explicitly to provide children with an opportunity—in an emotionally secure situation—to 'work through' their experience. A number of examples of such programmes are discussed in Tolfree's book *Restoring Playfulness* (1996).

Understanding of the process of socialisation is key in planning effective psychosocial intervention with children. Ager (1995) has suggested the model of Figure 10.1 to appraise both the impact of displacement and experience of conflict on a child's conceptualisation of the world, and of the means to foster (re)adjustment. The child's developing understanding of the world is seen to be influenced by direct experience, experience mediated through the family (e.g. accounts of parents) and experience mediated through wider social structures (e.g. instruction and modeling through the school, church or mosque).

In the course of war and displacement these very channels of socialisation by which the child makes sense of the world are disrupted, impairing their capacity to assimilate new experience in their understanding. This may be particularly critical when a child encounters violence or disruption which is outside the realm of their previous experience, and thus expectation. This child's understanding of their world—their 'map'—no longer fits with their direct experience, and the mechanisms by which sense can be made of this experience are impaired. In such circumstances not just the restoration of previous mechanisms of social learning, but also specific 'mediating' experiences to help assimilation of experience (including therapeutic use of songs, pictures and play), may be valuable (Richman 1993).

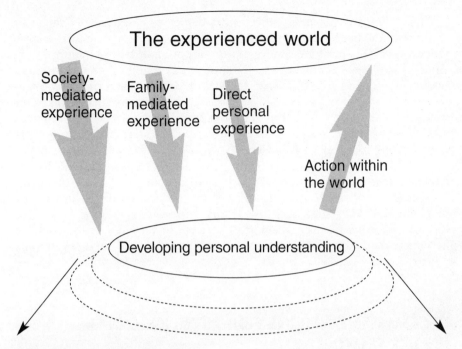

Figure 10.1 Model of influences on a child's developing understanding of the world (after Ager 1995)

Social Anthropology

While a number of the above theoretical approaches support the value within psychosocial interventions of strengthening and, where necessary, rebuilding community resources, it is social anthropologically informed critiques of psychosocial programming (e.g. Bracken, Giller and Summerfield 1995; Summerfield 1999) which have articulated most strongly the importance of appraising indigenous constructions of the impact of displacement. There is a clear danger that interventions framed in terms of assumed universal responses to events marginalise local, indigenous understandings of psychosocial need. This is not just a matter of the political 'good' of involvement of potential beneficiaries in programme planning. At a pragmatic level, there is a good deal of evidence of the ineffectiveness and/or inappropriateness of interventions which have been developed in this manner (Harrell-Bond 1986, 1999; Summerfield 1999).

A number of writers have noted the potential importance of integrating indigenous healing rituals and similar activities within psychosocial programmes, but the work of Wessells and colleagues in Angola is one of the few examples of this being followed through in intervention practice (Wessells 1998). Nonetheless, there does appear to be an increasing sensitivity within programmes of explicitly relating goals and methods to local belief, expectation and priority.

Thus while the preceding theoretical perspectives suggest a range of strategies for working with refugees such as Mrs Mukandori, frameworks used to plan assistance and support need to be sufficiently flexible—and those utilising them sufficiently humble—to ensure that her own priorities and perceptions are key determinants of the form of support she receives. It is easy to give 'lip service' to such respect for indigenous understanding, but the power differentials between refugees and those offering assistance are commonly so wide that active steps need usually to be made to ensure that a coercive form of relationship is not established (Harrell-Bond 1999). Such active steps may usefully include refugee representation within project management and evaluation, establishment of advocacy schemes and the facilitation of the previously noted mutual assistance networks. More generally, there is a clear case for seeing means of strengthening the 'voice' of refugees in the contexts in which they find themselves as a major priority of any programme which seeks psychosocial impact.

RECOMMENDATIONS FOR PSYCHOSOCIAL PROGRAMMING

While the previous section has noted the diverse theoretical perspectives which influence contemporary approaches to psychosocial intervention with refugee populations, there is—across such programmes—an increasing acknowledgment of some of the key characteristics which represent 'best practice' within the field. In 1996 the Task Force on Refugees and Forced Migration of the European Federation of Professional Psychologists Associations produced a report documenting such practice with respect to the four phases of the refugee experience noted earlier. That report sought to identify key features of best practice for a broad audience of policy makers, governmental officials and health and social welfare professionals. What follows is a revision of this analysis, tailored particularly to the agendas of those working in fields where promoting the psychosocial well-being of refugees is a key goal, though it still may be of value in briefing wider audiences on key issues.

The guidelines focus on the specific actions that may be appropriate in support of refugee psychosocial adjustment at various stages of the refugee experience. The emphasis is generally on social, educational and consulting actions potentially within the core remit of those working to promote psychosocial well-being in refugee populations. However, it is crucial to acknowledge the parallel and supportive role played by material and economic assistance in all these circumstances. Support for housing, employment, access to appropriate nutrition and household goods etc. are practical measures with huge potential impact on psychosocial well-being.

Appropriate Forms of Response in Emergency Situations

Greater awareness of—and sensitivity towards—the various stresses during the phases of forced migration can help agencies assist displaced persons, asylum-seekers and refugees more effectively. This will often not only be in the best interests of such assisted persons, but will also commonly support the efficiency and effectiveness of the agency itself. This is nowhere more the case than in emergency situations where agencies may be dealing with large numbers of disorientated and physically frail refugees.

Briefing of Personnel

It is important that humanitarian assistance workers, registration officers and others involved in working with refugees in emergency situations have a basic understanding of the psychosocial stresses commonly experienced during forced migration. In addition, such workers should also be made aware of the value of family integration, kinship support, cultural routines and practices etc. which can play a vital role in sustaining displaced persons coping capacity. Conflict management skills are also likely to be of significant value to front-line workers in emergency circumstances.

Cultural Mediation and Technical Assistance

There is considerable evidence that cultural mediation is a key component of successful management of emergency refugee situations. Technical assistance—whether with respect to psychosocial need or other concerns—needs to be 'brokered' through individuals with knowledge of the language, values and concerns of the refugee community. Identification—and empowerment—of representatives of the refugee population who can assist in this function is a crucial precursor to the effective deployment of any technical expertise regarding emergency psychosocial programmes.

Community Development Emphasis

Even (perhaps especially) in emergency situations, a community development emphasis needs to be brought to any psychosocial assistance offered. An emphasis on maintaining (or re-establishing) cultural forms and meanings is likely to prove of more sustainable value than individually orientated interventions which are frequently alien to cultural practice. Such principles should inform general assistance planning. For example, the planning of accommodation can respect family and ethnic grouping. The literature also strongly supports an emphasis on family reunification and temporary fostering schemes rather than 'orphanage' provision for unaccompanied minors.

Appropriate Responses with Asylum-seekers

Briefing of Personnel

Briefing of personnel involved in the assistance of asylum-seekers (including those processing asylum applications) can play a key role in avoiding unnecessary anguish for refugees. As above, it may also assist agencies in being more effective in their work. While conflicts between asylum-seekers and various components of 'officialdom' are inevitable, the successful management of such conflict can be promoted through a greater awareness of the stresses of the asylum-seeking process, and the basis of common reactions to them.

Provision of Counselling

The pressures of 'living in limbo' during an extended period of asylum are so common that the provision of some form of counselling support during this phase should be the norm. Such counseling provision may appropriately range from information giving regarding the processes of asylum application to forms of psychological support (including, in a minority of cases, formal psychotherapy). The range of such available supports should be clearly communicated to asylum-seekers.

Facilitation of Informal Networks and Befriending

Coping with the stresses of asylum-application, and longer-term adjustment for those resettling in a country of asylum, is supported by the availability of social resources. While professional input may be of value, social networks are a key indicator of psychosocial adjustment. Facilitation of asylum-seeker support networks among co-ethnic applicants can provide valuable solidarity during a difficult time. Befriending networks which 'bridge' an asylum-seeker into local indigenous population groups can support longer-term community integration.

Psychology and Asylum Decisions

In some circumstances professional psychological judgement may be requested regarding an asylum application. This will typically be in relation to an assessment of an applicant's claim regarding their 'well-found fear' of circumstances in their country of origin. In requesting such input agencies should establish the experience and expertise of the professional in dealing with clients from other cultures who have been exposed to traumatic events. Agencies should also acknowledge the ethical guidelines within which professional psychological practice should be conducted.

Appropriate Responses with Resettling Refugees

Addressing Acculturation Issues

Adjusting to a new culture provides a major challenge for many resettling refugees. Social and economic forces within countries of asylum frequently force refugees to the margins of society. Children 'mainstreamed' into society through state schooling may typically integrate within the host culture far more quickly than other members of their family, creating conflicts within the family. School, health and employment services should be orientated to the special needs of resettling refugees. All such services should be aware of specialist agencies which can be called upon to assist them in the fulfillment of their responsibilities to clients of their services who happen to be refugees.

Empowerment of Mutual Assistance Networks

While professional and voluntary agencies may play this supporting role in helping refugees adjust to life in a new country, mutual assistance networks (networks of refugees for refugees) show considerable promise in easing transitional stress. Such agencies may be of particular value in assisting refugees retain a sense of historical and cultural identity during the process of acculturation within a host society.

Professional Psychological Support

Evidence suggests that a proportion of resettling refugees are likely to benefit from psychological intervention of an appropriate form. This may be to assist in the management of acculturative stress, but may relate also to psychological distress with its origins in traumatic experiences during the pre-flight or flight phase. Refugees may also have existing and enduring mental health needs that require support.

Prompt identification of those suffering acute distress is important in ensuring timely intervention. Social support, community development, re-establishment of cultural forms and routines etc. will often form the 'first line of defence' with respect to psychosocial needs of many individuals. However, direct therapeutic work is likely to be of particular value when either such supports are not able to be put in place or—having been put in place—have been shown to be ineffective in resolving distress. For such clients referral to generic health and/or social services will normally be appropriate in the first instance.

Appropriate Responses with Repatriating Refugees

There is relatively little evidence regarding factors influencing psychosocial adjustment on repatriation. However, based upon the little work that has

been done—and general principles generated from related areas of work—
two major issues of potential relevance can be identified.

Facilitation of Family and Community Contact

Supporting repatriating refugees in re-establishing contacts with their families and communities will serve to reduce the disorientation experienced by
returnees following extended exile. Such contacts have clear social value,
but by commonly assisting also in the re-establishment of economic liveli-
hood, provide broader indirect support for psychosocial well-being.

Anticipation of Acculturative Stress

While reconnecting with existing social networks clearly supports a refugee
returning to their home country, refugees frequently experience considerable adjustment difficulties with regard to the changes that have taken place
in their absence. This suggests that agencies working with returnees should
be sensitive to the issues of acculturative stress in an exactly analogous
fashion to that commended above for refugees resettling in a country of
asylum. Both preparation of returnees prior to return, and their support
during the period in which they are re-establishing.

IMPLICATIONS

We close by returning to the situation of Mrs Mukandori. What does the
preceding analysis and, in particular, the recommendations above suggest
would have been valuable interventions to support the psychosocial well-
being of herself and her family?

Such a question again reinforces the complexity and multi-factorial nature
of psychosocial needs—it is apparent that no single intervention is likely to
have transformed the course of Mrs Mukandori's experience. But there are a
number of points—and levels—at which intervention may have (and may
still) impact the degree of her distress and suffering. Mrs Mukandori has
been faced with many officials and assistance workers since her first displacement, and any sensitivity that they may have shown with respect to an
understanding of the psychological dimensions of uprooting would have
been beneficial. Work of local or international agencies in Rwanda or former
Zaire supporting documentation of separated families and, potentially, the
exposure of human rights violations, may have played a useful preventive
function. Clearly resources targeted to protection and support of Rwandan
refugees crossing into former Zaire may have impacted Mrs Mukandori's
decision making regarding flight from the region—and the resultant separation from her remaining family. It was noted earlier how statistically excep-
tional Mrs. Mukandori is in the respect of her flight to the developed world.

The majority of women in Mrs Mukandori's position remain (or perished) in the region, and political, social and economic aid targeted at the fabric of society remains a likely foundation for psychosocial recovery of individuals and communities. Forms of counselling provision, within this broader context, may prove valuable. Such support for Mrs Mukandori, on either side of the Rwandan border, may have assisted in life-shaping decisions about flight and family.

On arrival in Canada Mrs Mukandori benefited from psychological counselling and medical care, but there were few facilities to support her with respect to acculturative stresses. Mutual assistance networks, ethnic associations or befriending groups may all have played a useful role here, in addition to support that would usefully be provided by the state in supporting settlement. Practical support in the areas of housing and employment also stands to provide people such as Mrs Mukandori with opportunities to bolster psychosocial well-being, as well as economic viability.

Finally, if resolution of Mrs Mukandori's situation is seen in terms of her being reunited with her children, then the role of efficient and effective communication regarding family members cannot be underestimated. Further, as she plans to be reunited with them—either by repatriating to Rwanda herself or by seeking consent from the immigration authorities for them to join her in Canada—she faces a complex political and legal bureaucracy. Any support for her in navigating such complexities promises to serve as a powerful psychosocial intervention.

REFERENCES

Adjukovic, D. and Adjukovic, S. (1998) *Trauma Recovery Training: Lessons Learned*. Zagreb: SPA.

Ager, A. (1995) Children, war and psychological intervention. In S.C. Carr and J. Schumaker (Eds) *Psychology and the Developing World*. New York: Praeger.

Ager, A. (1997) Tensions in the psychosocial discourse: implications for the planning of interventions with war-affected populations. *Development in Practice*, 7(4), 402–407.

Ager, A. (1999) Perspectives on the refugee experience. In A. Ager (Ed.) *Refugees: Perspectives on the Experience of Forced Migration* (pp. 1–23). London: Pinter.

Ager, A., Ager, W. and Long, L. (1995) The differential experience of Mozambican refugee women and men. *Journal of Refugee Studies*, 8(3), 263–287.

Agger, I. (1995) *Theory and Practice of Psycho-Social Projects Under War Conditions in Bosnia-Herzegovina and Croatia*. Brussels: ECHO.

Agger, I. (1997) *The Blue Room: Trauma and Testimony Among Refugee Women—A Psycho-Social Exploration*. London: Zed Books.

Agger, I. and Mimeca, J. (1996) *Psycho-Social Assistance to Victims of War in Bosnia-Herzegovina and Croatia: An Evaluation*. Zagreb: ECHO/ECTF.

Ahearn, F., Loughry, M. and Ager, A. (1999) The experience of refugee children. In A. Ager (Ed.) *Refugees: Perspectives on the Experience of Forced Migration* (pp. 215–236). London: Pinter.

Berry, J.W. (1992) Acculturation and adaptation in a new society. *International Migration*, 30, 69–83.

Bracken, P., Giller, J. and Summerfield, D. (1995) Psychological responses to war and atrocity: the limitations of current concepts. *Social Science and Medicine*, 40, 1073–1082.

Callamard, A. (1999) Refugee women: a gendered and political analysis of the refugee experience. In A. Ager (Ed.) *Refugees: Perspectives on the Experience of Forced Migration* (pp. 194–214). London: Pinter.

Doná, G. & Berry, J. (1999) Refugee acculturation and re-acculturation. In A. Ager (Ed.) *Refugees: Perspectives on the Experience of Forced Migration* (pp. 169–195). London: Pinter.

Harrell-Bond, B. (1986) *Imposing Aid*. Oxford: Oxford University Press.

Harrell-Bond, B. (1999) The experience of refugees as recipients of aid. In A. Ager (Ed.) *Refugees: Perspectives on the Experience of Forced Migration* (pp. 136–168). London: Pinter.

Joseph, S., Williams, R. and Yule, W. (1997) Understanding Post-Traumatic Stress: A Psychological Perspective on PTSD and Treatment. Chichester: Wiley.

Kinzie, J.D., Boehnlein, J.K., Leung, P.K., Moore, L.J., Riley, C. and Smith, D. (1990) The prevalence of post-traumatic stress disorder and its clinical significance among Southeast Asian refugees. *American Journal of Psychiatry*, 147, 913–917.

Kinzie, J.D. and Sack, W. (1991) Severely traumatised Cambodian children: research findings and clinical implications. In F.L. Ahearn and J.L. Athey (Eds) *Refugee Children: Theory, Research & Services* (pp. 92–105). Baltimore, MD: Johns Hopkins University Press.

Kraus, H. (1939) Starting life anew in a strange country. *Annals of the American Academy of Political and Social Science*.

Krupinski, J., Stoller, A. and Wallace, L. (1973) Psychiatric disorders in east European refugees now in Australia. *Social Science and Medicine*, 7, 31–49.

Loughry, M. and Ager, A. (1999) *The Refugee Experience: A Psychosocial Training Module*. Oxford: Refugee Studies Programme.

Majodina, Z.Z. (1999) The re-entry adaptation of returning South African exiles. Unpublished doctoral dissertation, University of Cape Town.

Marsella, A.J., Bornemann, T., Ekblad, S. and Orley, J. (1994) *Amidst Peril and Pain: The Mental Health and Well-being of the World's Refugees*. Washington, DC: APA.

McCallin, M. (1996) *The Psychological Well-Being of Refugee Children: Research, Practice and Policy Issues* (2nd edn). Geneva: International Catholic Child Bureau.

Mollica, R.F. (1994) Southeast Asian refugees: migration history and mental health issues. In A.J. Marsella, T. Bornemann, S. Ekblad and J. Orley (Eds) (1994) *Amidst Peril and Pain: The Mental Health and Well-being of the World's Refugees* (pp. 83–100). Washington, DC: APA.

Mollica, R.F., Donelan, K., Tor, S., Lavelle, J., Alias, C. and Frankel, M. *et al.* (1993) The effect of trauma and confinement on functional health and mental health status of Cambodians living in Thailand-Cambodia border camps. *Journal of the American Medical Association*, 270(5), 581–586.

Mollica, R.F., Wyshak, G. and Lavelle, J. (1987) The psychosocial impact of war trauma and torture on Southeast Asian refugees. *American Journal of Psychiatry*, 144, 1567–1572.

Muecke, M.A. (1992) New paradigms for refugee health problems. *Social Science and Medicine*, 35, 515–523.

Murphy, H.B.M. (1955) Refugee psychoses in Great Britain: admissions to mental hospitals. In H.B.M. Murphy (Ed) *Flight and Resettlement* (pp. 173–194). Paris: UNESCO.

Ressler, E.M., Boothby, N. and Steinbock, D.J. (1988) *Unaccompanied Children*. New York: Oxfor University Press.

Richman, N. (1993) Annotation: children in situations of political violence. *Journal of Child Psychology & Psychiatry*, 34(8), 1286–1302.

Summerfield, D. (1999) Sociocultural dimensions of war, conflict and displacement. In A. Ager (Ed.) *Refugees: Perspectives on the Experience of Forced Migration* (pp. 111–135). London: Pinter.

Tolfree, D. (1996) *Restoring Playfulness: Different approaches to assisting children who are psychologically affected by war or displacement*. Stockholm: Radda Barner.

Van der Veer, G. (1998) *Counselling and Therapy with Refugees and Victims of Trauma* (2nd edn). Chichester: Wiley.

Westin, C. (1999) Regional analysis of refugee movements: origins and response. In A. Ager (Ed.) *Refugees: Perspectives on the Experience of Forced Migration* (pp. 24–45). London: Pinter.

Zetter, R. (1999) International perspectives on refugee assistance. In A. Ager (Ed.) *Refugees: Perspectives on the Experience of Forced Migration* (pp. 46–82). London: Pinter.

Chapter 11

Designing Sustainable Health Promotion: STD and HIV Prevention in Singapore

George D. Bishop and Mee Lian Wong

Sexually transmitted diseases (STDs) have plagued humankind since time immemorial and the advent of AIDS, beginning in the 1980s, has served to considerably heighten concerns about their spread (Lewis, Bamber, and Waugh 1997). Singapore is no exception in this respect (Yeoh 1997). Rates for STDs, such as syphilis and gonorrhoea, have fluctuated greatly over the years with overall rates most recently peaking in the late 1970s at more than 950 cases per 100 000 population annually before dropping in the mid-1990s to less than 200 per 100 000 population (Ang and Chan 1997). This rate is still a matter of concern and the appearance of AIDS has inevitably added to those concerns. A small island with a population of 3 million, Singapore is situated in South-East Asia, a region with established epicentres for the AIDS epidemic.

Despite its proximity to Thailand, Cambodia, and other countries with high rates of HIV infection, Singapore has thus far had a relatively low rate. As of the end of 1998, 930 Singaporeans were reported to have been infected with HIV since 1985 when the first case of HIV was detected (Lim 1999). Of these, 311 have died leaving 619 living individuals with HIV/AIDS for an overall prevalence rate of 19.4 per 100 000 population. Of those infected, approximately 90% are male. Although the first cases of HIV were reported among homosexuals, since 1990 the preponderance of HIV infections have been contracted through heterosexual contact, with many apparently coming from sex with prostitutes. Given the close proximity to established

Cultivating Health: Cultural Perspectives on Promoting Health. Edited by M. MacLachlan.
© 2001 John Wiley & Sons Ltd.

epicentres for the epidemic and Singapore's small size, as well as the mobility of its population, a major challenge has been to keep the HIV infection rate low (Chew *et al.* 1991). As the spread of STDs and AIDS has been associated with commercial sex work, a major focus of attention has been on reducing the rate of STDs in sex workers and keeping them free of HIV (Wong *et al.* 1992). Critical questions, however, are how can this be accomplished and how can infection rates be kept low among other groups as well?

CASE STUDY

DO I HAVE THE RIGHT TO ASK CLIENTS TO USE CONDOMS?

Ms Tan is a 25-year-old registered female brothel-based sex worker in Singapore with nine years of schooling. She has been in prostitution for only four months. Three months ago, she was found to have cervical gonorrhoea during her monthly screening for sexually transmitted diseases at the Department of STD Control. She has been advised by the clinic nurse to use condoms with all her clients. She, together with her peers, has also attended a talk on the complications and dangers of STDs and AIDS and the effectiveness of condom use. She was also taught the proper technique on how to put the condom on the penis.

One month ago, Ms Tan was re-infected with cervical gonorrhoea. The doctor who treated her found that she was well informed about the seriousness of AIDS and STDs and the effectiveness of condom use. She then asked her why she did not use condoms even though she knew about their effectiveness. She gave the following reply:

> 'Do I have a right to ask the client to use a condom? He is paying me for my service and I have no right to demand from him. If I ask him to use condoms, he may get angry with me and I would lose my client to my peers. Besides, he may complain about me to the brothel keeper and I may even lose my job! Of course I want to protect myself. I am afraid of getting AIDS. But what can I do? I asked a client once to use a condom. He got angry and asked me why he should use a condom and whether I suspected him of having AIDS.'

Ms Tan is probably one of the many inexperienced sex workers who have encountered similar problems. This case study clearly illustrates that having knowledge of the seriousness of STDs and AIDS does not in itself lead to the adoption of safer sexual practices. Thus programmes aimed at condom promotion to prevent HIV or STDs among sex workers must go beyond information dissemination to addressing the other issues influencing condom use. These include affecting attitude change, increasing self-efficacy of the sex workers, equipping them with negotiation skills, mobilizing support from brothel keepers and peers, and targeting education programmes at clients themselves.

CENTRAL ISSUES

The control of STDs and HIV raises a number of important issues, particularly as it relates to commercial sex work. First, commercial sex in Singapore is a highly stigmatized activity. Singaporeans pride themselves on their promotion of family values and express overwhelming disapproval of commercial sex and of men seeking the services of prostitutes (Heng *et al.* 1992; Kok *et al.* 1995). As is the case in many countries, prostitution is illegal and there has been an ongoing debate over the years over the best approach to controlling of STD infection, and more recently HIV, as spread through prostitution (Yeoh 1997).

The current approach can best be described as one of 'harm reduction' in which brothels are allowed to operate but sex workers are required to participate in the Medical Surveillance Scheme, established in 1976. Brothel-based commercial sex workers are required to undergo monthly laboratory and clinical examination for gonorrhoea and chlamydia and quarterly screening for syphilis and HIV. Sex workers found to be infected with STDs are treated and prevented from plying their trade until such time as they are shown to be STD-free. Those found infected with HIV are prevented from continuing with their trade and deported if they are not citizens. This scheme is enforced with the help of the Anti-Vice Unit of the Singapore Police Force, which works closely with the Department of STD Control (DSC) of the Ministry of Health to ensure that brothel keepers send their sex workers for their regular screenings. The Anti-Vice Unit is empowered to suspend sex workers from their work, de-register them from the medical scheme, and deport them to their home countries if the sex workers do not comply with screening or treatment (Wong, Chan and Koh 1998; Yeoh 1997).

Second, the behaviour involved in the spreading of STDs and AIDS is very private. Sex workers are generally visited surreptitiously and the interaction which can lead to the transmission of STDs or HIV takes place out of the view of other persons. As such there is no practical way of verifying the nature of the interactions and whether condoms were used, other than through self-report or whether one of the participants contracts an STD. More importantly, whether condoms are used for sex may often be a matter of negotiation between the sex worker and client. Surveys of sexual attitudes and behaviour have found that clients visiting sex workers often resist suggestions to use condoms and frequently do not use them (Bishop, Kok and Chan 1998; Heng *et al.* 1992; Wong *et al.* 1994a). Thus an important aspect of any intervention programme is likely to involve motivating sex workers to make fundamental changes in their interactions with clients. Specifically such changes should enable them to protect their health by increasing their control over their sexual behaviours and lives, sometimes called 'empowerment'. Also it is essential to create a supportive working environment to facilitate safer sexual practices such as consistent condom use.

Third, for any intervention to be effective in reducing STD and HIV transmission it must be sustainable. Changes towards safer sex practices are always to be desired but to be truly effective in reducing the transmission of STDs and HIV in the long term they must be sustained over time. There have been a number of studies showing short-term reductions in risky behaviour (Ford *et al.* 1996; Geeta *et al.* 1995; Williams *et al.* 1992) but few evaluating their long-term sustainability (Asamoah-Adu *et al.* 1994; Visrutaratna *et al.* 1995). Thus we know that sexual practices of sex workers can be changed in the short term but this is really only the first step. Maintaining that change is a much more difficult challenge for controlling STDs and HIV. For example, an intervention with sex workers in Ghana increased consistent condom use from 6% to 71% after six months but this increase was not fully sustained, decreasing to 56% after 4 years (Asamoah-Adu *et al.* 1994).

THE CULTURE OF SEX WORK IN SINGAPORE

Commercial sex in Singapore, as elsewhere, is very complex. Sex workers in Singapore work from a number of venues including the streets, brothels and bars. Our focus here is on sex workers in brothels as they are the most easily identifiable and are under the Medical Surveillance Scheme. The case of non-brothel-based sex workers will be discussed later. To address the issues outlined above it is essential to have a detailed understanding of commercial sex workers and their problems and needs. This includes information on their psychosocial concerns and felt needs; their health needs such as the prevalence of STDs, AIDS and HIV infection and risk factors for their occurrence; the cultural and psychosocial factors governing their working conditions; their working environment; and determinants of their behaviour such as knowledge, beliefs, attitudes, values and self-efficacy. In other words, it is essential to understand what might be called the culture of brothel-based sex work in Singapore.

This requires both qualitative and quantitative methods. To address the issues raised several different methods were used to assess the circumstances and needs of brothel-based commercial sex workers in Singapore. To begin with, an epidemiological study was conducted on 806 brothel-based sex workers in 1990 to determine the incidence of STDs and their risk factors (Wong *et al.* 1992). The overall STD incidence rate in 1990 was 47.7 per 100 sex workers per year. The risk of STDs increased with number of clients and decreasing condom use. Sex workers who reported condom use with less than 40% of their clients were 2.13 times more likely than consistent condom users (100% condom use with clients) to develop STDs. Next, a survey on knowledge, attitudes and risk behaviours of the brothel-based sex workers found that the majority (>90%) were well informed of the seriousness of HIV and AIDS, the modes of transmission, and the effectiveness of condom use and were thus keen to use condoms (Wong *et al.* 1994a). However, they succeeded only half the time in getting clients to use them. Perceived barriers and low self-efficacy, rather than lack of knowledge, were found to be related to the lack of condom negotiation and low success in getting clients to use condoms. However, a minority of the sex workers claimed that they were able to get all their clients to use condoms.

This preliminary work helped to identify important areas for STD prevention and health promotion and also to obtain insights into the psychosocial circumstances of sex work and the interactions which sex workers have with their clients. Key areas identified for intervention included helping sex workers to overcome barriers to condom negotiation and developing their condom negotiation skills. However, this still did not provide in-depth information on their problems of condom negotiation or how to develop their negotiation skills. The next phase of the needs-assessment strategy thus focused on using qualitative methods to answer these questions. In-depth interviews were held with 40 sex workers with a wide range of success in condom negotiation in order to obtain a broad representation of their perceived barriers and approaches used (Wong *et al.* 1994a). The main reasons for not using condoms with clients were found to be lack of confidence in requesting clients to use condoms, and lack of negotiation skills to respond to clients' difficult queries and psychological pressure. For example, they did not know how to respond to the following questions from their clients: 'I am not afraid of death. Why are you afraid? If you are afraid, you should not work in this line'/'Why do you want me to use condoms? Do you suspect me of having AIDS?'/'Why do you want me to use condoms? Do you have AIDS?'

Overall they identified four groups of difficult clients: the young unmarried care-free client who does not think about the repercussions of not using condoms; the older client with no family responsibility and who does not worry about dying from AIDS, the regular client who trusts the sex workers and does not see the need to use condoms and those who cannot function with condoms. Other important barriers to condom negotiation included fear of losing clients to their peers and annoying brothel keepers who might see them as being fussy and thus not recommend clients to them.

However, there were some sex workers who succeeded all the time in getting clients to use condoms. In-depth interviews were held with them to help identify some successful approaches to negotiating condom use. The approaches that worked appeared to vary considerably and could be categorized into the positive, assertive, fear arousal and peer pressure approaches. Some examples of these approaches are as follows. Sex workers who used the *positive approach* made clients see the immediate benefits of condom use by telling them that 'condoms help them last longer' or that they have a wife and children to support. With the young unmarried client, the sex worker would remind them not to jeopardize their bright future or potential by contracting AIDS from non-condom use. The more experienced sex workers would use the *fear-arousal approach* by explaining to clients the dangers of AIDS and conveying their vulnerability to it:

'My previous client looks dirty and unwell. I am not sure whether he has spread AIDS or STDs to me. You better use a condom to protect yourself.'

The following approach was commonly used if clients should query whether they have AIDS:

> 'Regular tests do not show I have AIDS but one can never tell whether I have got AIDS after my recent test. My last client could spread AIDS or STD to me. For your own good, you better use a condom.'

Some sex workers would use the *assertive approach* to override difficult situations posed by clients:

> 'If my client challenges me as to why I am scared of dying, when he is not, I will tell them "Yes, I am scared of dying because I still have children to support. If you want to die from AIDS you go ahead but please do not drag me into it".'

Invariably this works and they agree to use condoms.

The less aggressive but more experienced sex workers used peer pressure to influence their clients. Some also used the concept of government policies to put pressure on them to use condoms. 'Most of my clients use condoms nowadays. You better use them too.' 'The government is spending a lot of money putting these posters up because AIDS is a serious problem now. You better use a condom.'

In summary, the data from these preliminary studies helped to identify areas for intervention which included equipping sex workers with negotiation skills; helping them overcome barriers to condom negotiation, and gathering support from brothel keepers and peers. It also helped to develop appropriate health education messages and materials that met the needs of the sex workers.

MODELS OF HEALTH PROMOTION

The next step in developing an intervention is the development or selection of a theoretical model (or models) for guiding the intervention. Not all health-promotion programmes are successful in achieving their objectives and there is substantial evidence from the literature on health promotion to suggest that the use of theoretical frameworks or models will significantly improve the chances of success in achieving pre-determined programme objectives. The use of models can help us understand better the nature of the problem being addressed, the needs and motivations of the target population, and/or the context for intervention, thus helping to achieve a better fit between problem and programme.

A number of models have been developed to guide ways in which we could bring about individual behaviour change, community actions, health supportive organisational practices and more effective communication of health messages for action. The models can be categorized into the following:

(1)   Models focusing on *individual behaviour change* such as the health belief model (Strecher and Rosenstock 1997), theory of reasoned action (Montano, Kasprzyk and Taplin 1997), stages of change model (Prochaska, Redding and Evers 1997) and social learning theory (Baranowski, Perry and Parcel 1997).

(2)   Models that focus on *mobilizing the community* to positively influence health such as community mobilisation (Minkler and Wallerstein 1997) and diffusion of innovation (Oldenburg, Hardcastle and Kok 1997).

(3)   Theories that guide the use of *communication strategies* for change to promote health such as communication for behaviour change (Egger, Donovan and Spark 1993) and social marketing (Andreasen 1995).

(4)   Models that focus on creation of health supportive *organizational practices* such as theories of organizational change (Goodman, Steckler and Kegler 1997) and models of intersectoral action (O'Neill, Lemieux and Groleau 1997).

(5)   Models focusing on development and implementation of healthy *public policy* such as ecological framework for policy development (Milo 1987).

(6)   *Overarching approaches* which attempt to integrate insights from other models into an overall framework for intervention such as Green's PRECEDE–PROCEED Framework (Green and Kreuter 1991). This is a comprehensive framework that combines many theories together into one model. It stresses identifying target group needs first such as various educational, behavioural, organizational and environmental factors influencing their health before planning and evaluating a health-promotion programme.

   As behaviour is very complex, being influenced by multiple factors, there may well be no single theory or model which can adequately guide the development of a comprehensive health-promotion programme intended to influence the multiple determinants of health in populations. Practitioners and policy makers are likely to need to draw on several theories or models, besides using local knowledge and experience, and available research information to assess the target group or community needs and the determinants of health which are most amenable to change at any particular time.

   After examining available models three were selected as providing the most insights and as being most likely to lead to a successful and sustainable intervention. These models were Green's PRECEDE–PROCEED framework (Green and Kreuter 1991), Bandura's self-efficacy theory (Bandura 1986) and the theory of reasoned action (Ajzen and Fishbein 1980; Montano, Kasprzyk and Taplin 1997).

   The PRECEDE–PROCEED framework was selected as a systematic integration of different theoretical approaches to health promotion so as to provide a structure for applying various theories in developing appropriate interventions. As such the PRECEDE–PROCEED framework can be thought of as a 'road map' for negotiating the various hurdles to effective behaviour change. Specifically, this framework identifies nine phases for a successful health education intervention (see Figure 11.1). The PRECEDE phases involve diagnosis of the problem at the social, epidemiological, behavioural and environmental, educational and organizational, and administrative and policy levels. This diagnosis then leads into the PROCEED phases which include the health-promotion effort itself followed by evaluation of the process, impact and outcome of the intervention. Throughout these phases detailed attention is given to the variety of factors that influence the health and quality of life of the population involved. As such this 'road map' provides a comprehensive approach to understanding the myriad factors involved in the problem and its solution.

Using this framework, we identified condom negotiation as a changeable and important behaviour for intervention. First, sex workers were motivated to negotiate condom use by relating safe sex to what they value. The majority of them were in prostitution out of economic necessity to support family members. As such, the message stressed the money saved from being free of STD and AIDS. As noted above, all brothel-based sex workers are required to have frequent gonorrhoea tests. Testing positive for gonorrhoea would result in financial costs incurred from payment for medications, and a loss of earnings due to suspension from work.

Second, training was provided to equip them with negotiation skills to counter clients' arguments and develop assertive behaviour. Approaches used by their peers who succeeded in getting clients to use condoms were disseminated to them by means of talks, video presentations and printed materials.

Third, a supportive environment to facilitate behaviour change was provided by getting brothel keepers to display posters and remind clients to use condoms, and to encourage their peers to always negotiate condom use or refuse unprotected sex if the negotiation process fails.

In addition to this overall approach two more specific models were also applied. In particular, Bandura's social learning theory (Bandura 1986) and the theory of reasoned action (Ajzen and Fishbein 1980; Montano, Kasprzyk and Taplin 1997) were applied subsequently to maintain behaviour change. In his social learning theory Bandura argues that a key factor in people's behaviour is the belief they have about their ability to perform a specified behaviour, what he calls self-efficacy. It is not enough to simply know about the behaviour and know one should engage in it. One must also believe in one's capability to do so. As a key barrier to negotiating condom use appeared to be a low sense of self-efficacy among the sex workers for being able to negotiate successfully, interventions were developed to raise their self-efficacy. Bandura points out that one can increase a person's confidence in carrying out a task by getting her to observe or hear from friends who have done it successfully. Along these lines video presentations were developed demonstrating a sex worker successfully persuading different types of clients to use condoms or suggesting alternatives should the negotiation fail.

Next, the complexities of the target behaviour can be broken down into components that are relatively easier to manage. Using this theory, the act of

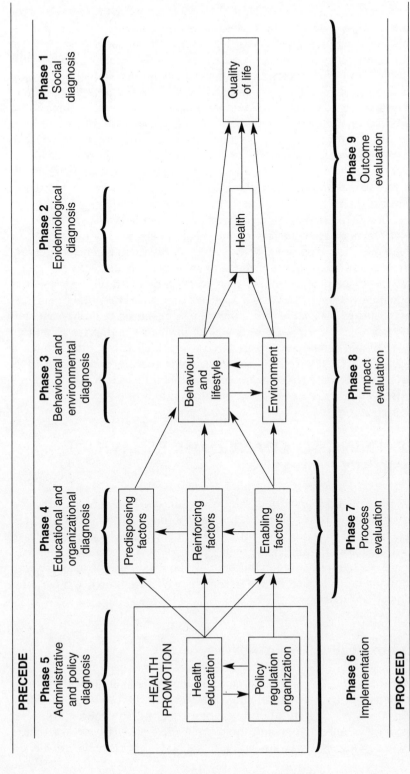

Figure 11.1 The PRECEDE–PROCEED model (after Green and Kreuter 1991: 24). Reproduced with permission of Mayfield Publishing Company

condom negotiation was divided into the non-verbal initiation stage and the negotiation stage. The first task was to use visual cues such as placing condoms at an easily visible place, for example near the pillow or wash basin, or displaying posters on condom use on the walls to prompt the client. If the client did not respond to the visual cues, the sex worker would then initiate negotiation by giving a condom to the client and telling him of the benefits of condom use. This would lead to compliance among some clients. With non-compliant clients, the sex worker was taught to anticipate questions and queries from them so that she could respond confidently with a counter-argument and assert her rights. If the client still refused to use condoms she would proceed to suggest alternatives such as massage or helping him to masturbate. Should this process also fail, she would refuse to take him as a client.

The theory of reasoned action proposes that the intention to act depends on subjective normative beliefs about what others think one should or should not do. Thus in the later phase of the intervention, when about three-quarters were using condoms, a message was promoted stressing condom use as the norm. Non-condom using sex workers would thus feel pressured to change if they did not want to face social disapproval from their peers. At this stage Bandura's social learning theory was also used to build their self-confidence, improve their skills to deal with problems arising from condom use and reinforce behaviour change. This was achieved by getting them to meet regularly in small groups to share problems, receive encouragement by hearing about the positive experiences of others and model each other's success in dealing with problems specific to condom use.

INTERVENING TO CHANGE RISK BEHAVIOUR AMONG SEX WORKERS

The intervention itself included four main phases. These were: first, the training of health-care providers in the environmental and behavioural approach to STD/HIV control; second, discussions with the brothel keepers to learn about their views and enlist their support; third, the interventions for the sex workers to encourage condom use; and, finally, the maintenance phase designed to evaluate the programme as well as reinforce and perpetuate the behaviour changes.

Training of Health-care Providers

Health facilitators (advisors) working at the public STD clinic were trained in the behavioural and environmental approach to STD/HIV/AIDS control. Training consisted of five 2-hour sessions covering the following areas: theories of behaviour change and their application; strategies to assess and change sex workers' behaviour; and methods and media in health education. The course was task oriented and stressed experiential learning and problem solving. Short lectures were given to deliver the basic principles and these were followed by case study discussion of actual problems identified from needs-assessment studies, practical exercises, role-playing and simulation learning. A handbook was developed and given to participants for easy reference. The nominal group process technique was used to get health facilitators to work collectively and prioritise problems and possible solutions for action.

Group Discussion with Brothel Keepers

Group discussions were held with brothel keepers to encourage them to support sex workers in condom negotiation and refusing sex without a condom. They were also requested to remind clients to use condoms. Discussion was highly interactive and focused on possible solutions to problems raised by them. Some brothel keepers expressed their inability to control the negotiation process between the sex workers and their clients. They were assured that skill development sessions would be conducted for sex workers to increase condom use among them. Brothel keepers were also reminded of the benefits of an STD-free brothel and checks by the Department of STD on their compliance to support sex workers in condom use.

Interventions for Sex Workers

The next phase of the programme was the interventions with the sex workers themselves. In designing these interventions it was essential to take careful account of various cultural factors influencing the sexual practices of the sex workers, their perception of vulnerability to AIDS and STDs and their attitudes towards condom use. For example, the anus is perceived by many of the local Chinese and non-Chinese sex workers as a dirty, shameful, excretory organ, which may explain the fact that less than 2% practised anal sex. Also some of the sex workers had fatalistic beliefs and felt that using condoms would not make a difference in protecting them if they were destined to be a prostitute and to get AIDS. Further, many of the sex workers in Singapore are in prostitution to support their families. Many of them shared common cultural values of putting their children or families before self and see prostitution as a source of steady income to provide for their families. Thus messages to the sex workers that relate condom use or safer sex to these values were found to be effective in motivating them to negotiate condom use with their clients. For example, sex workers were told to use condoms to prevent AIDS so that they could continue to work to support their families and not get AIDS that would bring suffering to their families.

In training sex workers to negotiate with clients it is also important to take account of the cultural values of clients. The majority of the clients in

Singapore are local Chinese with the others being foreign workers from other Asian countries, expatriates from both Asian and Western countries, and tourists. For clients culturally relevant messages linking safer sex to family values and not bringing shame or 'loss of face' proved to be effective. For example, sex workers often found the following approach to be effective:

> 'You should use a condom so that you will not get AIDS or STDs. What will your family members think of you if they know that you have AIDS from having sex with me, a prostitute? You will make them "lose face". Surely, you do not want to be a burden to your family.'

With these considerations in mind, interventions for sex workers were aimed at motivating them to negotiate condom use, developing their negotiation skills and increasing their assertiveness in refusing sex without a condom. The following basic messages were delivered: (1) always use condoms; (2) you have a right to refuse sex and protect yourself from STD and AIDS; (3) regular clients are not safe; and (4) no one loses and everyone is a winner if all cooperate.

Groups of about 16 sex workers were organized to provide a heterogeneous mix of sex workers with differing attitudes and skills in condom negotiation so as to get them to share their individual polarized views and experiences and provide support to each other under the encouragement and guidance of a health facilitator. Each group was given two 2-hour skills training sessions and a booster session.

The objectives of the first skill development session were to get sex workers to know each other better, clarify their values and misconceptions, and to demonstrate, by means of the video, practical ways of getting clients to use condoms. The video presentations consisted of six short video clips in which volunteers among the sex workers role played common problem situations. The video clips (running time of 3 minutes per clip) covered the following topics:

(1) First week at work
(2) Persuading a young client to use condoms
(3) Regular clients need persuading too
(4) How about a massage?
(5) You have the right to refuse
(6) A healthy woman's advice

- *First week at work.* This clip shows an inexperienced sex worker getting advice from her seniors on condom use and her rights to safe sex.
- *Persuading a young client.* This clip shows the use of a positive approach to persuade a young client. The sex worker tells the client he has potential and a bright future ahead and one day he would like to get married and have children. She then emphasizes the point that it is not worth dying from AIDS as a result of not using condoms.

- *Regular clients need persuading too.* An older regular client is persuaded to use condoms in this clip. The old client refuses to use condoms because he trusts the sex worker to be 'clean' as she is screened regularly for STDs. The sex worker then explains that she cannot tell whether her last client has passed STD or AIDS to her and she has asked him to use condoms for his own protection. The client is not convinced and responds that he does not worry about dying from AIDS as he has no family responsibility. The sex worker follows with a counter-argument that one does not just die from AIDS but suffers a great deal from it. She also integrates community cultural values into the message by telling him he may lose 'face' and bring suffering and shame to his family. She then reassures him that he will not lose sensation with the use of condoms. The client finally agrees to use condoms.
- *How about a massage?* This clip depicts a situation where a client refuses to use condoms in spite of all the persuasion. The sex worker then suggests a massage to which the client agrees at a discounted rate.
- *You have a right to refuse.* This clip shows a sex worker with a resistant client who refuses condoms and other alternatives. The sex worker politely refuses to take him as a client and returns his money. The client then storms out of the room. The sex worker remains cool, accepting it as part of her work.
- *A healthy women's advice.* The last clip shows a sex worker persuading her peers to cooperate and use condoms or refuse sex without a condom. She stresses peer unity and cooperation to fight for their rights against unsupportive brothel keepers and resistant clients.

Each video clip presentation was followed by a discussion of other problems they had experienced and possible solutions. Many sex workers asked for support from the health facilitators to talk to brothel keepers. Sex workers also role-played to increase their self-efficacy and to practise assertive behaviours. They were subsequently asked to keep, for three days, a log book of clients who refused to use condoms with regard to their reasons for not doing so and the difficult queries posed by them when asked to use condoms. This self-monitoring exercise was to increase the sex workers' awareness of what they were doing, which was a starting point for gaining control.

During the second session, health facilitators led the group to discuss problems in persuading clients to use condoms arising from their self-monitoring of condom use. The experienced peers gave practical tips on how to deal with difficult clients. Sex workers were also given posters (stating 'condoms must be used here') for display in their brothel-rooms to facilitate their negotiation task (see Figure 11.2).

Three months later, a booster session was held with distribution of free condoms and comic scripts depicting common problems encountered with clients and their solutions. A comic book was designed in an entertaining form that sex workers like to read. Focusing on personal experiences of the sex workers, it was meant to reinforce the video clips and group discussions. It depicts a story of a sex worker, Mei Ling, who meets her friend Alice at a

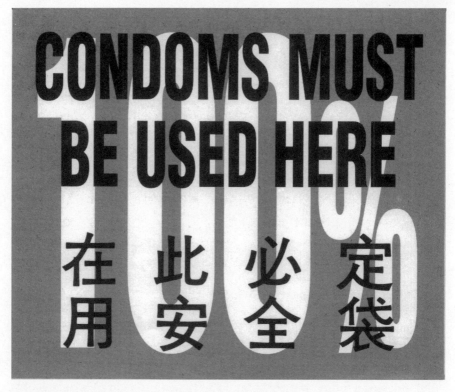

Figure 11.2   Posters displayed in brothels (after Wong *et al.* 1992: 413). Reproduced with permission of Baywood Publishing Company, Inc.

public STD clinic. Alice has gone there for a gonorrhoea injection. Mei Ling, the more experienced sex worker encourages her to use condoms by telling her the benefits. Alice raises many doubts and problems to which Mei Ling provides practical advice and answers. Alice subsequently tries the approaches that Mei Ling has suggested and finds them not too difficult after all. The story thus ends with Alice, the younger sex worker, gaining self-esteem. Selected scenes from the comic book are shown in Figure 11.3.

Maintenance Phase of the Project

The maintenance phase consisted of three follow-up problem-solving sessions held 6 months to a year apart. Regular meetings were held with peer leaders to get feedback on problems encountered and discuss possible solutions. Some problems encountered after the initial phase were non-supportive brothel keepers who recommended clients to non-condom-using sex workers; acceptance by some sex workers of clients that were refused by their peers for not using condoms; decrease in clients because of condom use; and increased self-reports of condom slippage, breakage, pain, and clients' complaints of failure to ejaculate from condom use. The peer leaders

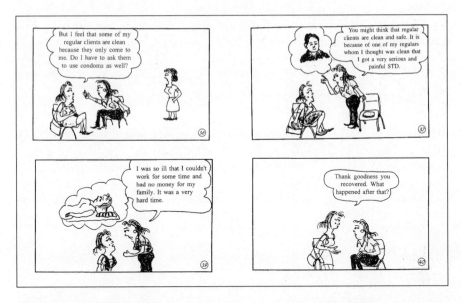

Figure 11.3 Sample from comic script (after Wong *et al.* 1992: 415). Reproduced with permission of Baywood Publishing Company, Inc.

proposed that the Anti-Vice Unit take action on non-compliant brothel-keepers. The Department of STD control thus held meetings with the Anti-Vice Unit and got their cooperation to act on non-compliant brothel keepers. Brothels found recommending clients to non-condom-using sex workers were given warnings, and those with high gonorrhoea rates were temporarily suspended from business by the Anti-Vice Unit.

The second author also acted promptly to provide individual counselling to non-condom-using sex workers that were made known to her by the peer leaders. Sex workers in the programme had learned from their clients who the non-condom-using sex workers were. The stages of behaviour change model (Prochaska, Redding and Evers 1997) was applied to assess the sex worker's readiness to use condoms and identify their reasons for not using condoms so that advice could be matched to their needs.

During the follow-up sessions, sex workers shared practical tips on how to deal with problems such as condom slippage, condom breakage, clients' failure to ejaculate from condom use and pain from prolonged condom use. Early adopters of consistent condom use also reassured their peers that the initial decrease in clients was temporary, as many of their former clients returned and agreed to use condoms.

After one year, when about three quarters of the sex workers were always refusing unprotected sex, the message was reinforced that it was a norm to use condoms so that non-compliant sex workers were pressured to change their behaviour. Compliant sex workers were also encouraged to persuade their non-condom-using peers to use condoms and to share their positive experiences and coping strategies with them. The continual interest and commitment of health staff to the programme were obtained by giving them frequent feedback on the project and involving them in discussing problems and developing solutions.

Evaluation of the Project

Evaluation of the project was accomplished in two ways. First, *impact and outcome evaluation* was performed by comparing the behaviours and gonorrhoea rates of 124 sex workers receiving the intervention with those of 122 demographically similar sex workers in a control group. Second, *process evaluation* was accomplished through interviews with sex workers concerning their experiences during the programme and perceptions of the intervention and its success.

Impact and Outcome Evaluation

Evaluation of the impact and outcome of the intervention was assessed by comparing behaviours at baseline with those at five months, one year, and two years post-intervention and by comparing the gonorrhoea rates among sex workers for the five months before the intervention with those for the five months post-intervention. Following the five-month evaluation the control group was no longer retained for ethical and administrative reasons and the intervention was given to all sex workers. Full details of the design for this evaluation are given elsewhere (Wong *et al.* 1996; Wong, Chan and Koh 1998).

The results of this evaluation showed that the intervention had been highly successful both in changing behaviour and in reducing gonorrhoea rates. As can be seen in Table 11.1, sex workers receiving the intervention showed considerable improvement in negotiation skills, with the mean success rate in getting clients to use condoms rising from 66.1% at baseline to 80.2% at 5 months. The proportion of those who always refused sex without a condom increased considerably by 20.8% from 44.4% at baseline to 65.2% at five-month follow-up. These changes were corroborated by a significant 77.1% reduction in the five-month cumulative gonorrhoea incidence from 10.5 per 100 persons to 2.4 per 100 persons in the five-month period before and after intervention. The control group only showed an improvement of 3.7% in negotiation skills and there was no change in behaviour outcomes of refusing unprotected sex. Gonorrhoea incidence in the control group decreased by 37.6%. However, this result was statistically non-significant and may be the result of chance factors.

The intervention group was then followed up regularly for two years. The changes were maintained at two-year follow-up with negotiation skills increasing to 91.1% and consistent refusals of unprotected sex increasing to 90.5%. Gonorrhoea incidence declined to 1% over the same period. These changes are shown in Figures 11.4 and 11.5.

Table 11.1 Behaviour and gonorrhoea rates at baseline and five months post-intervention. Wong *et al.* 1998: 896. Reproduced with permission of Academic Press, Inc., Orlando, Florida 32887-6777

Outcome	Control group (n = 122)	Intervention group (n = 124)	Observed rate ratio[a] (95% CI)	Adjusted rate ratio (95% CI)
Average success rate[b] in persuading clients to use condoms (%)				
Preintervention	68.4	66.1		
Postintervention	71.6	80.2		
Observed difference	3.2	14.1		
No. (%) always refusing sex without a condom				
Preintervention	49 (40.2)	55 (44.4)	1.10 (0.75–1.62)	–
Postintervation	37 (35.2)[c]	72 (65.2)[c]	1.85 (1.25–2.76)	1.90 (122–2.94)[d]
No. (%) with gonorrhoea				
5-month period before intervention	24 (19.7)	13 (10.5)	0.53 (0.27–1.05)	–
5-month period after intervention	15 (12.3)	3 (2.4)	0.20 (0.06–0.68)	0.21 (0.06–0.73)[e]

[a] Observed rate ratio is the ratio of percentage always refusing sex without a condom or gonorrhoea incidence rate in the intervention group to that in the control group.

[b] The average success rate refers to the mean of the success rates of all the sex workers in that group. The success rate of each sex worker refers to the reported proportion of clients of 10 who used condoms following negotiation.

[c] Excludes missing responses. There are 17 missing responses in the intervention group and 14 missing responses in the control group for this question.

[d] Adjusted rate ratio of percentage always refusing sex without a condom that is adjusted for baseline percentage and race and age of the sex workers using Cox regression model modified for cross-sectional data.

[e] Adjusted rate ratio of gonorrhoea rate that is adjusted for race and gonorrhoea rates at baseline by modification of Cox's model.

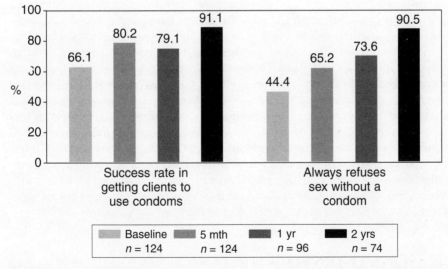

Figure 11.4 Change in negotiating skill and condom use (after Wong *et al.* 1998: 897). Reproduced with permission of Academic Press, Inc., Orlando, Florida 32887-6777

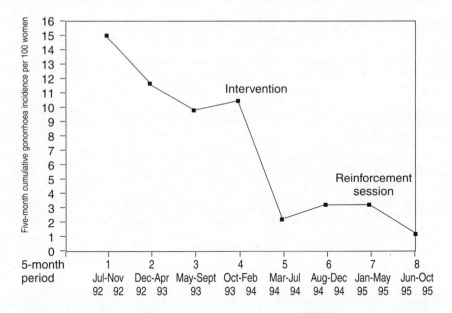

Figure 11.5   Changes in gonorrhoea rates (after Wong *et al.* 1998: 898). Reproduced with permission of Academic Press, Inc., Orlando, Florida 32887-6777

Process Evaluation

Evaluation of the process leading to behaviour changes was accomplished through in-depth interviews with 22 randomly selected sex workers two years after the intervention. Several reasons were cited for their success in increasing condom use. Among these were the effectiveness of the negotiation techniques learned, the use of the posters with the message '100% condom use: condoms must be used here', and learning techniques to prevent condom slippage, breakage and pain. The sex workers also reported that their fears about a reduction in the number of clients had proven unfounded and that even though the numbers had initially declined they later returned to normal. In addition, their confidence was reinforced when former clients returned and agreed to use condoms. Finally, condom use had become easier over time as clients accepted the norm of condom use. In fact, all 22 sex workers interviewed reported that they did not even need to negotiate condom use with clients about a year after the intervention as they had developed the confidence and skills to put the condom on their clients without even asking them as the clients had already accepted that as the normal procedure.

LESSONS LEARNED

This project very clearly demonstrates the feasibility and effectiveness of behavioural and environmental interventions to promote health and reduce gonorrhoea among brothel-based sex workers. Several studies have shown that STDs facilitate the transmission of HIV and a clinic-based intervention consisting of STD control and condom promotion can help in preventing HIV/AIDS (Wong 1995).

Even though this project was specifically targeted at sex workers in Singapore there are several lessons that can be drawn from it and applied in settings with other populations and cultural groups. First, an essential aspect of this project was the use of a comprehensive health-promotion model that applies principles and theories from the behavioural, social and management sciences to promote positive health behaviour, in this case safer sex practices among sex workers. The use of the PRECEDE–PROCEED framework as well as Bandura's self-efficacy formulation and the Theory of Reasoned Action helped to identify critical areas for examination and ultimately behavioural intervention. Without the guidance of these theoretical formulations the efforts to alter behaviour would have been much more sporadic and, we believe, far less successful.

Second, it is important to examine the overall context of the behaviour in question and to intervene with groups who, even though they are not the main target of behaviour change, have a significant impact on the behaviour in question. Thus, even though our target group was sex workers, interventions were made with other groups such as brothel keepers and health staff to create a supportive workplace environment to facilitate behaviour change. For example, posters were displayed in all brothels to remind clients to always use condoms and brothel keepers were instructed to talk to clients about condom use and support sex workers in turning away non-compliant clients. In addition, the nominal group technique was used with the health facilitators to get their involvement and commitment in programme implementation and the Anti-Vice Unit of the Singapore Police Force was brought in to enforce compliance with health regulations.

Third, to be effective the intervention must address target group needs, which are best determined by a complement of quantitative and qualitative techniques, and must involve members of the target group, as well as relevant others, in the project formulation and the design of culturally relevant messages. In this project both qualitative and quantitative methods were used to make a careful assessment of the circumstances, behaviour, and beliefs of the sex workers and the sex workers themselves were involved in programme development and implementation. In addition, discussions were held with brothel keepers to obtain their input and get their support.

Finally, it is often useful to utilize a combination of intervention methods. In this case the use of a combination of health-education methods enabled us to meet the differing needs of the sex workers more effectively. The group approach was useful in sharing experiences and enlisting support, whereas individual counselling allowed the health educator to accommodate individual differences, assess the stage of change of the individual's behaviour and provide personalized advice. Similarly the use of both video clips and comic books made presentation of the message more effective in that the video clips dramatized the behaviours in a vivid fashion for the sex workers during training, whereas the comic books presented the message in a form that the sex workers enjoyed reading and could take away with them.

APPLYING THESE LESSONS TO OTHER CHALLENGES FOR THE CONTROL OF STD AND HIV

The approach described above has proven effective in changing behaviour and controlling gonorrhoea among brothel-based sex workers. How might the lessons learned be applied in changing behaviour and controlling STD and HIV in other populations? On the one hand, many of the details of this project may be able to be fairly directly adapted for use among brothel-based sex workers in South-East Asian communities and other communities with similar socio-cultural environments. On the other hand, for other groups the adaptation may need to be on a less direct and more conceptual level. For example, the intervention may not be directly replicable in other settings where street-based sex workers predominate. However, certain principles which contributed to the effectiveness of this project could be adapted for use in such settings: application of sound theory, use of a complement of quantitative and qualitative techniques to assess target group needs, multiple strategies, and participatory involvement of health-care providers and the target population in planning the interventions. In the next few paragraphs we consider some of the other challenges for the control of STD and HIV in Singapore and how the principles elaborated above might apply.

Streetwalkers

As noted earlier, commercial sex in Singapore is complex and involves more than just brothel-based sex workers. A group that is of concern but has only recently been targeted for intervention is sex workers who ply their trade from the streets, bars, and pubs. Streetwalkers and other freelance commercial sex workers in Singapore operate completely outside of the law and are not involved in the Medical Surveillance Scheme that covers brothel-based sex workers. They are a rather amorphous group, reputedly often foreigners, and speak a variety of languages. There is also reported to be a high turnover rate, particularly among the foreigners, and individual sex workers appear to have particular territories from which they solicit clients (Action for AIDS 1999).

As yet there has been little or no systematic study of freelance commercial sex work in Singapore, although popularized accounts exist (Brazil 1998). Currently the only intervention being implemented for this group to encourage safer sex practices is the Streetwalker Project being conducted by volunteers from Action for AIDS, Singapore's sole AIDS NGO (non-governmental organization). In this project volunteers go at night to locations where streetwalkers are known to ply their trade and distribute condoms and information booklets in various languages to the sex workers. Also informational lecture sessions on safer sex practices have been organized for the sex workers at locations accessible to them (such as rented hotel rooms in areas where they work) but these have had limited success, owing at least in part to the unwillingness of sex workers to cross each others' territories to attend the sessions (Action for AIDS 1999).

The challenges posed in changing behaviour in streetwalkers have both similarities and differences with the challenges posed by brothel-based sex workers. On the one hand, it would appear, at least on the surface, that some of the same materials and skill building techniques may be useable by both groups. On the other hand, the delivery and maintenance of the programme is likely to be somewhat different. First, the social structure of the sex work varies considerably between brothel-based and non-brothel-based sex workers. Among the factors which contributed to the success of the programme among brothel-based sex workers are the support that the programme received from the brothel owners and the efforts taken by the Anti-Vice Unit against non-compliant brothel keepers. This social structure is not available to reinforce the programme with streetwalkers. Rather the interventions, of necessity, will need to be targeted at the level of individual sex workers and without the assistance of outside agencies.

Since the activities of streetwalkers and other freelance sex workers are completely illegal and many of the sex workers may be foreigners with at best a tenuous immigration status, bringing in the Anti-Vice Unit would only serve to drive them further underground and thus further from the reach of the intervention. Another major difference with streetwalkers is the amorphousness of this group. As noted, this group is made up of both locals and foreigners and there is reportedly a high turnover among the sex workers. This suggests that interventions will need to be continuous to reach new sex workers as they begin work. In addition, language presents a problem in that the sex workers are likely to speak a variety of different languages and thus materials need to be in these languages in order to be effective. Finally, the dynamics of sex work are likely to be very different between the brothel and the street, suggesting that new approaches may well need to be developed in order to effectively reach streetwalkers.

At this point such considerations are highly speculative since as yet no detailed assessment has been made of streetwalkers and other freelance sex workers. Before effective interventions can be designed and implemented it is essential that such an assessment be made. This type of assessment was key in designing and successfully implementing the programme with brothel-based sex workers and a similar strategy can be utilized with streetwalkers.

Clients of Commercial Sex Workers

Thus far our attention has focused on sex workers in the fight against STDs and HIV. The other part of this equation is, of course, the clients of sex workers. As noted earlier, there is evidence that a significant number of men visiting sex workers use condoms inconsistently if at all (Bishop *et al*. 1998) and that efforts are needed to reduce risky sexual behaviour, especially with sex workers. One aspect of this is addressed through interventions with the sex workers. When sex workers successfully negotiate condom use this reduces the risk to the client. However, Singapore is a small country and it is not unusual for Singaporean men to visit sex workers in other countries where the sex workers may or may not insist on the use of condoms. As such there is a need for interventions to encourage safer sexual practices for men visiting sex workers regardless of whether those sex workers are in Singapore or abroad.

Currently the primary means for getting the safer sex message to clients and potential clients of sex workers is through media campaigns as well as through talks, seminars and other events aimed at the general public as well as at specific target groups, including outbound travellers (Cheah 1998). Media campaigns have evolved over the years and have taken a number of themes, generally emphasizing the risks of casual sex and the importance of abstinence (for singles) and fidelity (for married individuals) as the keys to prevention. The use of condoms as a preventive measure has been included in media campaigns since 1992 but has always been a secondary message. Evaluations of these campaigns have indicated a high level of awareness of the campaigns although no evidence is available concerning their effects on actual behaviour (Heng 1998). In addition to these general campaigns posters have been displayed at various exit points from Singapore and a booklet entitled *A traveller's guide to good heath* emphasizing the importance of avoiding risky sex has been distributed at the same exit points.

Changing high-risk behaviour among the clients of sex workers presents challenges different from those with the sex workers themselves. For one thing, clients of sex workers are likely to be more difficult to identify than the sex workers, particularly brothel-based sex workers. Sex workers are generally visited surreptitiously and at varying frequencies with some clients seeking the services of sex workers on a regular basis whereas others visit infrequently or perhaps only once. While it might be possible to identify clients coming to brothels, this is much more difficult when streetwalkers or other freelance sex workers are involved. This problem is compounded by the fact that it is not uncommon for Singaporean men to seek sex workers overseas while travelling, making their identification for intervention all the more difficult.

This difficulty in identifying clients suggests that intervention programmes will need to take a somewhat different approach. It is probably not realistic to do a detailed needs assessment of the type done with brothel-based sex workers nor to do intensive interventions with this population. Rather, more indirect approaches are probably more realistic. On the one hand, one can target clients when they visit sex workers. This was, in effect, done in the programme for brothel-based sex workers described earlier. By teaching the sex workers to negotiate condom use the behaviour of clients was changed. This, however, only reaches clients visiting brothel-based sex workers and the effects may be limited to those specific encounters. It remains to be seen whether similar results can be obtained with non-brothel-based sex workers and whether the changes in client behaviour generalize to other encounters. Further, targeting clients when they visit sex workers is completely unrealistic for reaching those visiting sex workers overseas. In this case mass media approaches are probably the only realistic means for intervention. At this point the key question is how mass media messages can be constructed and delivered so as to have the maximum impact on behaviour. Messages used thus far have tended to be rather general in nature and, while there is evidence that people are aware of them, there is no evidence as yet concerning their effectiveness in actually changing behaviour.

Men Having Sex with Men (MSM)

Although the majority of HIV infections in Singapore were acquired through heterosexual contact a significant minority have come about through homosexual or bisexual contact. Since the first cases were detected in 1985 approximately 15% of infections have been through homosexual contact whereas roughly 11% have been among bisexuals (Toh 1998). Available evidence also points to unsafe sexual practices among a significant number of gay and bisexual men. For example, a survey of sexual practices among men attending an anonymous testing site in Singapore found that of men indicating sex with only men, over 40% reported high-risk encounters (unprotected penetrative sex) whereas for men reporting sex with both men and women more than 70% indicated that they had engaged in high-risk activities (Bishop et al. 1998). Also evidence from a convenience sample of gay men in Singapore suggests that they are more likely to engage in unprotected anal sex with casual partners than are gay men in Sydney, Australia (Van de Ven et al. 1998). Although data from these two studies cannot be considered representative of Singapore gays and bisexuals in general, they do point to the need for interventions for reducing risky sexual behaviour.

To date, gay and bisexual men have not been specifically targeted in media campaigns in Singapore and the only organized intervention programmes have been conducted by Singapore's AIDS NGO, Action for AIDS. These have consisted primarily of social events in bars and clubs during which information about HIV and safer sex has been highlighted and distributed. In addition, Action for AIDS runs an anonymous HIV testing site and a phone counselling service through which safer sex information is distributed (Action for AIDS 1999). As longitudinal surveys of sexual behaviour among gay and bisexual men have not been carried out there is no real way to evaluate the effectiveness of these efforts in reducing risky sexual behaviour.

Developing and implementing effective interventions for encouraging safer sexual practices among gay and bisexual men presents a number of challenges. Homosexual activities are illegal in Singapore, punishable by

imprisonment, and many gay and bisexual Singaporeans are deeply closeted (Leong 1995; Ng 1999). There are few exclusively gay venues, such as
bars and clubs, although some bars and clubs do cater for a predominantly
gay clientele on certain nights. In addition, there are no overtly gay organizations that are officially recognized in Singapore which has strict laws with
respect to the registration of organizations and societies. These facts, along
with the social stigma associated with homosexuality, often make it difficult
to identify gay and bisexual men, particularly those who are closeted and/
or do not utilize gay venues or participate in informal gay-related organizations, and directly target interventions to them. Along these same lines
owners of venues that cater to gays are often reluctant to be identified as
such and to serve as distribution points for safer sex information.

Although the situation of gay and bisexual men differs radically from that
of brothel-based sex workers a similar general approach may be useful. One
of the first steps needs to be a detailed qualitative and quantitative study of
gay life and particularly gay sexual behaviour. Beginnings have been made
with this (Ng 1999) but much more needs to be done. To date, there is
limited quantitative data available on the sexual behaviour of gay and bisexual men (Bishop *et al.* 1998; Van de Ven *et al.* 1998) and little, if any, qualitative data. This type of information on gay culture and sexual behaviour in
Singapore is critical to provide the basis for developing effective and sustainable programmes. To be effective these programmes would need to be
developed by, or at least with the active participation of, members of the gay
community.

Although the details of such programmes would need to await the availability of these kinds of data, we can speculate on some of the features of
these programmes. First, venues attracting a gay clientele are emerging and
sustained efforts should be made to utilize these venues for educating gay
and bisexual men about HIV and safer sex practices. Second, the Internet is
likely to play a key role in safer sex education for gay and bisexual men. Ng
(1999) points out that the development of the Internet in Singapore has had a
substantial impact on the development of gay awareness and a sense of
community among gay men and that such vehicles as e-mail, Internet Relay
Chat (IRC), and gay-related websites and newsgroups now serve as important channels of communication for Singapore gays. Such vehicles make ideal
mechanisms for communicating information about AIDS and safer sexual
practices and, indeed, are already being used. Action for AIDS has a website
(http://www.afa.org.sg) with safer sex information, issues relating to HIV
and AIDS are discussed on gay-related newsgroups and there is a wealth of
information on HIV and AIDS readily available through overseas sites
aimed at the general population as well as specifically at gay and bisexual
men. Future interventions can take advantage of the information already
available and supplement it with creative uses of internet resources. For
example, a very creative campaign, entitled Victor Vancouver, utilized Internet resources for a successful safer sex intervention targeted at gay youth in
Vancouver, Canada (Allan and Borley 1997). Third, even though overtly gay
social organizations are not allowed to exist officially there are a number of

informal gay organizations that serve as both social outlets and as support for gay men. These organizations can be used as a channel for disseminating information about HIV and AIDS and encouraging safer sexual practices.

Although a number of avenues can be imagined for getting the message to gay and bisexual men, many of these are likely to be effective in reaching primarily men who self-identify as gay or bisexual and may not be effective in reaching those who engage in sex with other men but are not self-identified as gay or bisexual and/or do not frequent gay venues, belong to informal gay organizations or make use of gay internet resources. For such individuals mass media may be more effective. In this respect we would second Toh's (1998) call for the integration of issues related to MSM into the National AIDS Control Programme in Singapore and for MSM issues to be specifically raised in national AIDS campaigns.

CLOSING COMMENTS

In this chapter we have detailed a successful intervention with brothel-based commercial sex workers and shown how the underlying model can be used to varying degrees with groups that differ from the original target group with respect to their circumstances and needs. The PRECEDE–PROCEED framework seems ideal in this respect in that it does not specify interventions to be used but rather lays out a systematic procedure for identifying interventions that are likely to be effective for the group in question. As such it seems particularly well suited to the development of interventions that span different cultural groups as well as different subcultures within a particular society. The specifics of the interventions to be used will almost certainly differ as, for example, the use of comic books for sex workers but Internet resources for gay and bisexual men. However, the general principles should remain essentially the same.

REFERENCES

Action for AIDS (1999) *Annual report 1998*. Singapore: Action for AIDS.

Ajzen, I. and Fishbein, M. (1980). *Understanding Attitudes and Predicting Social Behavior*. Englewood Cliffs, NJ: Prentice Hall.

Allan, B. and Borley, S. (1997) Victor Vancouver: A multimedia health promotion and research campaign for gay youth. Paper presented at AIDS Impact: Biopsychosocial aspects of HIV infection. Melbourne, June.

Andreasen, A.R. (1995) *Marketing Social Change: Changing behaviour to promote health, social development and the environment*. San Francisco, CA: Jossey-Bass.

Ang, P. and Chan, R. (1997) Sexually-transmitted diseases in Singapore—Trends in the last two decades. *Annals of the Academy of Medicine, Singapore*, 26, 827–833.

Asamoah-Adu, A., Weir, S., Pappoe, M., Kanlisi, N., Neequaye, A. and Lamptey, P. (1994) Evaluation of a targeted AIDS prevention to increase condom use among prostitutes in Ghana. *AIDS*, 8, 239–246.

Bandura, A. (1986) *Social Foundations of Thought and Action*. Engelwood Cliffs, NJ: Prentice Hall.

Baranowski, T., Perry, C.L. and Parcel, G.S. (1997) How individuals, environments and health behaviour interact. In K. Glanz and M.L. Lewis (Eds), *Health Behaviour and Health Education: Theory, research and practice* (pp. 153–178). San Francisco, CA: Jossey-Bass.

Bishop, G.D., Kok, A.J. and Chan, R.K.W. (1998) Sexual practices among men attending an anonymous testing site in Singapore. *AIDS Care*, 10(Suppl. 2), S167-S178

Brazil, D. (1998) *No Money, No Honey! A candid look at sex-for-sale in Singapore* (4th edn). Singapore: Angsana Books.

Cheah, C. (1998) AIDS education in Singapore. Paper presented at AIDS Conference 1998: Facing the challenge in Singapore, Singapore, December.

Chew, S.K., Lee, H.P., Monteiro, E.H.A. and Sng, E.H. (1991) Human Immunodeficiency virus infection in Singapore—Containment strategies. *Annals Academy of Medicine, Singapore*, 20, 362–368.

Egger, G., Donovan, R. and Spark, R. (1993) *Health and the Media: Principles and practices for health promotion*. Sydney: McGraw-Hill.

Ford, K., Wirawan, D.N., Fajans, P., Meliawan, P., MacDonald, K.N. and Thorpe, L. (1996) Behavioural interventions for reduction of sexually transmitted disease/HIV transmission among female commercial sex workers and clients in Bali, Indonesia. *AIDS*, 10, 213–222.

Geeta, B., Lindan, C.P., Hudes, E.S., Desai, S., Wagle, U., Tripathi, S.P. and Mandel, J.S. (1995) Impact of an intervention on HIV, sexually transmitted diseases and condom use among sex workers in Bombay, India. *AIDS*, 9(Suppl. 1), S21-S30

Goodman, R.M., Steckler, A. and Kegler, M.C. (1997) Mobilising organisations for health enhancement: Theories of organisational change. In K. Glanz, F.M. Lewis and B.K. Rimer (Eds) *Health Behaviour and Health Education: Theory, research and practice* 2nd edn (pp. 287–312). San Francisco, CA: Jossey-Bass.

Green, L.W. and Kreuter, M. (1991) *Health Promotion Planning: An educational and environmental approach* (2nd edn). Mountain View, CA: Mayfield Publishing.

Heng, B.H., Lee, H.P., Kok, L.P., Ong, Y.W. and Ho, M.L. (1992) A survey of sexual behaviour of Singaporeans. *Annals Academy of Medicine, Singapore*, 21(6), 723–729.

Heng, V. (1998) Evolution of AIDS media campaign in Singapore. Paper presented at AIDS Conference 1998: Facing the Challenge in Singapore, Singapore, December.

Kok, L.P., Heng, B.H., Ong, Y.W., Ho, M.L. and Lee, H.P. (1995) How sexually permissive are Singaporeans? *Annals Academy of Medicine, Singapore*, 24, 679–684.

Leong, L.W.T. (1995) Walking the tightrope: The role of Action for AIDS in the provision of social services in Singapore. In G. Sullivan and L.W.T. Leong (Eds) *Gays and Lesbians in Asia and the Pacific: Social and human services* (pp. 11–30). New York: Haworth Press.

Lewis, M., Bamber, S. and Waugh, M. (1997) *Sex, Disease, and Society: A comparative history of sexually transmitted diseases and HIV/AIDS in Asia and the Pacific*. Westport, CT: Greenwood Press.

Lim, A. (1999) About 200 new HIV cases last year. *The Sunday Times (Singapore)*, 25, 28 March.

Milo, N. (1987) Making health public policy: Developing the science by learning the art: An ecological framework for policy studies. *Health Promotion*, 2, 263–274.

Minkler, M. and Wallerstein, N. (1997) Improving health through community organisation and community building. In K. Glanz and M.L. Lewis (Eds) *Health Behaviour and Health Education: Theory, research and practice* (pp. 241–269). San Francisco, CA: Jossey-Bass.

Montano, D.E., Kasprzyk, D. and Taplin, S.H. (1997) The Theory of Reasoned Action and the Theory of Planned Behavior. In K. Glanz and M.L. Lewis (Eds) *Health Behavior and Health Education: Theory, research, and practice* (pp. 85–112). San Francisco, CA: Jossey-Bass.

Ng, K.K. (1999) *The Rainbow Connection: The internet & the Singapore gay community*. Singapore: KangCuBine Publishing.

O'Neill, M., Lemieux, V. and Groleau, G. (1997) Coalition theory as a framework for understanding and implementing intersectoral health-related interventions. *Health Promotion International*, 12, 79–85.

Oldenburg, B., Hardcastle, D.M. and Kok, G. (1997) Diffusion of innovation. In K. Glanz and M.L. Lewis (Eds) *Health Behaviour and Health Education: Theory, research and practice* (pp. 270–286). San Francisco, CA: Jossey-Bass.

Prochaska, J.O., Redding, C.A. and Evers, K.E. (1997) The transtheoretical approach and stages of change. In K. Glanz and M.L. Lewis (Eds) *Health Behaviour and Health Education: Theory, research and practice* (pp. 60–84). San Francisco, CA: Jossey-Bass.

Strecher, V.J. and Rosenstock, I.M. (1997) The Health Belief Model. In K. Glanz and M.L. Lewis (Eds) *Health Behaviour and Health Education: Theory, research and practice* (pp. 41–59). San Franciscom, CA: Jossey-Bass.

Toh, P. (1998) Men who have sex with men, bisexual males. Paper presented at AIDS Conference 1998: Facing the Challenge in Singapore, Singapore, December.

Van de Ven, P., Bishop, G.D., Chan, R.K.W. and Koe, S. (1998) A comparison of HIV risk among gay men in Singapore and Sydney. Paper presented at the 12th World AIDS Congress, Geneva, July.

Visrutaratna, S., Lindan, C.P., Sirhorachai, A. and Mandel, J.S. (1995) Superstar and model brothel: Develop and evaluating a condom promotion program for sex establishments in Chiang Mai, Thailand. *AIDS*, 9(Suppl. 1), S69-S75.

Williams, E., Lamson, N., Elem, S., Weir, S. and Lamptey, P. (1992) Implementation of an AIDS prevention program among prostitutes in the Cross River State in Nigeria. *AIDS*, 6, 229–242.

Wong, M.L. (1995) Behavioural interventions in the control of human immunodeficiency virus and other sexually transmitted diseases—A review. *Annals Academy of Medicine, Singapore*, 24, 602–607.

Wong, M.L. *et al.* (1992) Theory and action for effective condom promotion: Behaviour intervention project for sex workers in Singapore. *International Quarterly of Community Health Education*, 15(4), 413–415.

Wong, M.L., Archibald, C., Chan, R.K.W., Goh, A., Tan, T.C. and Goh, C.L. (1994a) Condom use negotiation among sex workers in Singapore: Findings from qualitative research. *Health Education Research: Theory and Practice*, 9, 56–67.

Wong, M.L., Chan, R.K.W. and Koh, D. (1998) A sustainable behavioural intervention to increase condom use and reduce gonorrhoea among sex workers in Singapore: 2-year follow-up. *Preventive Medicine*, 27, 891–900.

Wong, M.L., Chan, R.K.W., Lee, J., Koh, D. and Wong, C. (1996) Controlled evaluation of a behavioural intervention and programme on condom use and gonorrhoea incidence among sex workers in Singapore. *Health Education Research*, 11, 423–432.

Wong, M.L., Wong, C., Tan, M.L., Ho, J.Y., Lim, R., Lim, S., Wan, S. and Chan, R. (1994b) Knowledge and sexual behaviour related to HIV and AIDS of female sex workers in Singapore. *Health Education Journal*, 53, 155–162.

Wong, M.L., Wong, T.C. , Tan, M.L., Ho, J.Y., Lim, S., Wan, S. and Chan, R. (1992) Factors associated with sexually transmitted diseases in Singapore. *International Journal of STD and AIDS*, 3, 323–328.

Yeoh, B.S.A. (1997) Sexually transmitted diseases in late nineteenth- and twentieth-century Singapore. In M. Lewis, S. Bamber and M. Waugh (Eds) *Sex, Disease, and Society* (pp. 177–202). Westport, CT: Greenwood Press.

INDEX

Compiled by Indexing Specialists, Hove, E. Sussex